Energy Meditation: Healing the Body, Freeing the Spirit

Energy Meditation: Healing the Body, Freeing the Spirit

In conversation with Master Yap Soon Yeong

by
Chok C. Hiew

toExcel
New York San Jose Lincoln Shanghai

Energy Meditation:
Healing the Body, Freeing the Spirit

In conversation with Master Yap Soon Yeong

Published by toExcel,
an imprint of iUniverse.com, Inc.

For information address:
iUniverse.com, Inc.

620 North 48th Street
Suite 201
Lincoln, NE 68504-3467
www.iUniverse.com

ISBN: 1-58348-579-1

Printed in the United States of America

Foreword

by
Master S. Y. Yap
Founder of CFQ Energy Healing

Getting to know Chok C. Hiew when he arrived in Penang, Malaysia in early 1992 was more than a coincidence. Someone gave me a pamphlet about a workshop on optimizing health and states of consciousness conducted by a Canadian psychology professor. I was quite skeptical, at first, as Western techniques did not appeal to me. Moreover, the workshop was not cheap! But strangely, I felt strongly that I should attend and was literally drawn to go by some unseen force. During the self-introductions, he showed much interest when I mentioned that I was a alternative medicine practitioner and traditional healer. He visited me at my healing center after the workshop ended. From Canada, he remained in contact with me making many long distance calls. Subsequently, on each of his annual Asian visits he made it a point to spend time in my Center. At first glance, this interest was baffling. He was born in Penang and has many relatives and friends here, but instead he spent the limited time he had with me.

Chok Hiew, besides being a researcher in health psychology, has a life-long interest in meditation, Eastern healing arts, and Qigong. His involvement in different healing systems and inquisitive explorations have taken him to remote corners of the globe and well qualify him as a master in energy and meditative healing fields. And yet, he displayed the curiosity of an innocent child, never failing to ask about how I worked, and pushing to understand clearly what I meant right to the tiniest clinical detail. At the Center, he observed my healing work with patients with the intensity of a detached researcher to ensure that nothing escaped his notice. He spoke to my clients and students and interviewed them at great length. He consistently probed deeply to see whether patients had recovered and to what degree. I can almost read the uppermost question he held in his mind, "Is CFQ good enough to deliver all that it promises?"

Three years later, in 1995, he invited me to his home in Fredericton, Canada to talk about meditation and healing at the local university, and conduct some healing work in the community. He also brought me, for the first time, to the United States to conduct similar workshops and healing.

Chok suggested that I should let more people know about my work and volunteered to write about it since my own practice and teaching at the Center left me no time. He completed an earlier spiritual biographic book, 'Tao of Goldbody Energy Healing,' an as yet unpublished work. I suggested that he work on another book with a less esoteric title and a more practical outlook on healing suggestions for the reader.

So, here we go, this book, "Energy Meditation: Healing the Body, Freeing the Spirit," one product of seven years of our association. An ancient saying goes like this, 'False knowledges are circulated in ten thousand books but the truth is contained in one sentence within a single volume.' I believe this book is far from the false ten thousand. The essence of the truth shared in this book is simply—Let go and relax. Finally, I refer you to Bodhidharma, who brought Zen Buddhism to the Far East without a single word in writing. His teaching is: Search into your Heart to discover your true self.

Preface

09/09/99: Year of Earth Rabbit

Spending a year in Japan, I wanted to pursue Eastern energy healing traditions but it was a strange beginning arriving in Hiroshima. American journalists have voted Hiroshima as the site of the most potent world event of the 20th Century when the awesome power of atomic energy unleashed obliterated Hiroshima and some 200,000 lives in a single cataclysmic explosion. This occurrence demonstrates that it is energy that matters in creation and in the destruction of all life. Yet, Hiroshima rose from the ashes like a phoenix, and has today become a memorial for world peace. Human resilience has healed its citizens and brought great heights of prosperity and achievements. One Hiroshima survivor is Sakyemune Sensei, an internationally respected Japanese psychologist. With Sakyemune's encouragement, the flow of ideas on the psychology of longevity, transcendence, and resilience were developed, presented in professional conferences, and swiftly published in psychological journals in Japan.

From Hiroshima, I was close to the orbit of a remarkable Eastern energy healer living in my birthplace in Malaysia. This is Qigong Master Yap Soon Yeong of Penang, and his original "CFQ" system of Eastern medicine and spiritual development based on Taoism and Buddhist healing practices. In a career as a full-time healer for the past fifteen years, Master Yap has been responsible for hundreds of astounding cures of deadly diseases and brain injuries so advanced that conventional medicine had given up on these dying patients. I found time between traveling to international conferences to stop over, meet, and converse with Master Yap in Penang, Malaysia. These conversations, presented in this book, dwelled on the practice and experiences of meditation and energy healing that elucidated the essential principles of rejuvenation to enable the self repair response to reverse disease, aging, and ultimately to transcendence.

After each of the five visits to see Master Yap I would return back to Japan. Toward the end of my residence in Hiroshima, I met with Sakyemune who I learned came from a 500 year-old lineage of Buddhist priests in Miyajima Island. When I first asked him about doctors, hospitals, and medical insurance in case I became sick in Japan, he brushed them off remarking firmly that I won't need them. "Resilience will take care of you." Later on, when I felt the pangs of social isolation living alone in Japan, Sakyemune said, "Your meditation will remove your sense of suffering."

Half in jest, Sakyemune repeated a question he asked earlier when I first arrived in Hiroshima, "And have you become enlightened?" To be enlightened is not something that can be directly achieved but is an effortless and totally relaxed state of perception of reality itself. Enlightenment is here and has never left our innermost Heart or being. To see the "One who Knows", the seeker simply wipes off the impure energies that cling on. In the experience of the Golden Sage, the instant that nurturance of Stillness is done, one becomes connected with Perfection and the boundless radiance of Nirvana shines through. But read on to discover how in the ensuing dialogues with Master Yap on radiant Goldbody energy.

Chok C. Hiew, Ph.D.
Fredericton, New Brunswick

Acknowledgments

"Search into your Heart to find the True self

Relax, let go, and radiate!"

To Master Yap Soon Yeong, CFQ energy healing founder and Goldbody Light meditation healer, who journeyed with me on the path of self discovery to meet my inner teacher—the One who knows.

Contents

Introduction

The roots of Eastern energy healing practices, in traditional oriental therapies, Qigong, and martial arts originate from the indigenous Taoism of ancient China and early oral Buddhist traditions transmitted from India. Taoism asserts that the origin of the Universe is energy, which has positive and negative charges as represented by the 'tai-chi' symbol. The two opposite cosmic charges create constant changes represented by the hexagram symbol as set forth in the ancient 'I-Ching' or Book of Changes, explaining that these changes give rise to a Universe of infinite variety in living and inanimate matter. Twentieth century modern physics identified two basic principles of Quantum Theory: All matter is energy, and all things are connected. Cosmic or pure energy occupies a mass that is hundreds of thousands of light years across. Given that the speed of light is 186,000 miles per second, pure energy has near infinite vastness. Buddhist thought asserts that the origin of the Cosmos is a formless Emptiness (sunyata in Sanskrit) that is comprised of boundless luminous energy. This "Empty" energy is the basic building block that in transformation creates matter. Reality is a magnificent, seamless Emptiness that is ineffable but full of a vibrant cosmic consciousness without beginning or end.

Energy healing, in practice, is a continual awareness and the experience of letting go. With sufficient letting go, the root causes of the body's illnesses are released to be healed and then the Spirit shines. To learn more, face-to-face interactions and a direct transmission of knowing from Master Yap who lives in Penang, Malaysia was needed. Opportunity arose while I was in Japan to participate in a series of international psychology conferences. I made it a point to visit and meet Master Yap on each occasion.

1

On the Energy Side of
Homo Sapiens

In Eastern thought, all matter is said to be transformed from cosmic energy by way of stepping down the velocity of vibrations. Life forms have sophisticated systems to readily absorb cosmic energy to enhance their growth and life-sustaining functions. In humans, the mind together with the five senses, when stimulated, automatically convert the fine cosmic energy from the stimulants to be absorbed into the whole organism. Master Yap explains, "Such external qi energy has a basic characteristic—it is 'inward-drawing' and when drawn into the body is 'upward suspending' as the absorbed energy accumulates within. Thoughts, emotions, trauma of emotional and physical origins, and memories from past stimulations also leave behind large amounts of residual energy, and are also major sources of these 'inward-drawing' forces."

The absorbed residual energy from the external stimulants is stored in the various force centers in the body that are referred to as tension forces or dense energy forces. The force centers located in the torso or main body include specific energy centers referred to as 'chakras' and also in the entire body such as in the joints and the body parts where they meet as well as in the organs of vital functions. Other sources of tension energy include damaged tissues because of strenuous physical activation; injuries, infections, and past surgery.

Master Yap further revealed that, "Properties such as muscle and joint stiffness, hardening of arteries, tissue deformation such as lumps and knots in the musculature, and also the wrinkling and folds of aging, are said to be caused by the continual build-up of accumulated tension forces. The formerly fine energy, once transformed into the body system, has become debased. Naturally healthy functioning and rejuvenation of the physical body become obstructed when the following biological systems are affected: blood circulation, waste removal, digestion and nutrient assimilation; transmission of nerve system impulses, communication of inter-body parts and organs, cell and tissue replacement. These system breakdowns lead to health problems, vulnerability to infections, and disease. Aging is another by-product as the 'decay' process sets in due to the same tension forces accumulated. Aging, therefore is considered as a precursor to disease."

For all diseases, the fundamental noxious agent is tension force accumulation that restricts the flow of life energy. Energy healing techniques, must be effective in tension or dense energy force removal. Master Yap, drawing from his practice of Qigong healing in oriental medicine, teaches an energy healing technique that he calls Chaoyi Fanhuan Qigong or 'CFQ'. The energy technique "unwinds, melts, and releases the inward-drawing dense energies and tension forces within and without the body that are responsible for every kind of illness, disease, as well as aging. The CFQ energy approach is an anti-disease and anti-aging technique, as it dissolves and flushes out their one root cause—accumulated tension forces."

According to energy healer Master Yap, inherent self-healing as well as energy transmission to heal others is a skill that requires many years of practice to develop. The practitioner first learns how to clear out his or her own dense energy forces, even before symptoms of disease manifest. CFQ tunes into the tension forces and clears them out where they are strongest, primarily in the body's torso:

a) The base of the neck to hip section-accumulated mainly from physical origins,

b) The heart to head section—accumulated mainly from mental origins (emotions, thoughts, and psychosocial trauma).

Problems in one section affect other sections of the body. All problems including those in other regions(such as the limbs) can be traced to the main body, and can be dealt with by dealing with the latter. All these forces are linked to a common center—the energy heart (located around the heart) and which often result in an energy congestion in the chest region and vulnerability to disease. The detrimental effect of accumulated tension forces can be seen, by the trained CFQ healer, as a compacting effect on the body. There is a shortening of the muscles and tendons mentioned in a) and b) above. The most severely affected is the overlapping section of both areas, that is, the neck to heart sections. This also results in the formation of horizontal bands of tension forces. Overall, as in aging, cells and tissues glue together, harden, and shrink accelerating cell decline, decay, disease, and death.

Another effect is an uneven force distribution, as physically observable between the left and right side of the torso; and between the front and back of the body. They produced uneven, complicated tension patterns which affect the normal functions of the organs and muscles. For example, when accumulated tension hardens and compresses one side of the neck region, cerebral blood flow is imbalanced that can build up to cause a stroke.

The Meaning of Tao Energy

Traditionally, the term qi from Taoism meant energy, but then had different terms for different types of energy. Contemporary Qigong practice does not clearly state what type of qi is acquired during training. CFQ is concerned with healing by bringing through formless, boundless cosmic energy, and not more impure forms of qi energy. The Taoist word for cosmic energy is 'khun-yen qi.' Also the CFQ cultivation of radiant consciousness or Goldbody energy-state is a purification practice to best return to cosmic consciousness.

There is a special reason why the Ancients use the word qi, for energy instead of any other word. Qi is the same word that means 'air'. In the advanced stage of meditation, the body becomes so relaxed that one is no longer confined to the physical body, so that one cannot even find the boundaries of the physical body. One is simply part of everything, the cosmic, and totally free. That free state, in ancient times, had no word to describe it. The closest equivalent is air, that is free and unrestricted.

Qigong has been misinterpreted and misunderstood today and people think of it as the art of understanding breathing and learning how to breathe. The incorrect belief taught is that the purpose of Qigong is to, 'absorb the pure energy from air.' True practice, however, is not about learning how to breathe, or how to absorb the essence from air. Rather, Qigong describes the art of attaining the state of ultimate relaxation and the purpose is to be 'as loose as thin air.' One is so relaxed, and so free as to be bodiless and weightless, so that one does not even have a physical body.

Scientific reports have described the measurement of qi energy in terms of electromagnetic fields. But in line with CFQ, the body energy that is measured here also has impurities. Certain Eastern martial training methods can certainly strengthen such fields in the body. But again, the CFQ principle is not to consciously try to strengthen, as it is letting go of weaknesses that is crucial. For example, a weakness, problem, or disease area in the body often has a stronger magnetic field than a healthy one. So a strong field measured does not necessarily mean that a person is healthier. What is most important is the dynamics of the field, i.e., that the energy must flow properly.

Cultivating the Tao

Master Yap explains the significance of meditation as an energy balancing and grounding technique to rejuvenate and prevent disease:

"CFQ, is a method of cultivating total relaxation and stresses simplicity in method. It means that CFQ does not apply complex concepts in practice theorized in traditional oriental therapy such as 'yin' and 'yang', the five elements, and meridians. Related to the notion of simplicity, CFQ meditation is an effortless approach, in terms of understanding energy, by using minimum mental effort, without using strong visualizations, or any rigorous method. When the body is totally relaxed, it balances itself into a state of perfect health."

"The dense energy forces form into energy fields within the body and around us. The energy fields connect us to animate and inanimate objects outside our body, so that the connection leads to mutual influence. As such, the attached energy forces, that form one component of our physical body, store the seed or cause of future events—this is the law of causation that is commonly referred to as 'karma'. "

Karma is a Sanskrit term for actions—of body, speech, and mind, and all such actions produce subtle energy seeds which in time will spawn further consequences. Karma is an Eastern notion commonly used to explain the differing conditions of the world. For instance, people enjoy good health and pleasant life circumstances as a consequence of good deeds performed in the past in one's present lifetime and perhaps previous lives, for karma is a force that survives death.

Master Yap asserts that CFQ meditation can remove the karmic forces that have become physically attached to us. Therefore, we are not only able to overcome and reverse life span problems such as our illnesses and aging, but the purified energy patterns also influence the social environment positively. We also change our current and future life circumstances for the better. Tension forces are a form of debased energy and to remove them, one must bring in the energy of relaxation. Biological and psychological methods of cognitive-behavioral relaxation, including intentional visualizations, are external or 'acquisition methods' that cultivate mental energy which have a residual tension component. Mental energy is karmic by nature since it is generated by the mind and attaches to the body. All such methods cannot be effective in complete removal of impure energies and tensions.

Master Yap explains the essence of CFQ this way:

"Relax and you will be fine. Those are words you most often say to others and hear others say to you in times of trouble. In fact, these words slip out of our mouths without much thought. But how often did our troubles get solved by just relaxing? Indeed, it should always be! But then few of us actually think that troubles can be solved this way. Often people mouth these words because they cannot offer an alternative suggestion. I beg to disagree. Relaxation really works!"

"What precisely is relaxation? Is it about doing nothing at all? Just go and sleep our troubles away? Take a holiday? Sweat and burn it off? Simply have a good time out? Or just forget about them?"

"Well, it's none of the above! You actually have to do something in order to relax. You actually have to be courageous. You need to go right in and come face to face with the energy source of the trouble, melt it off, and literally free it out. Then the actual problem does go away. At least the pain or mental agony is removed. But it is effortless relaxing and bravery."

CFQ attempts to cultivate true relaxation by means of a non-acquiring or letting go method. Dense energy or detrimental forces that have accumulated in the body are unwound, melted, diluted, and flushed downwards. There is an opening outwards of the released tension from the entire person. The body is kept relaxed, soft and loose, letting go of all physical and mental tensions. The lower abdomen is the center of awareness (not concentration, as it generates mental energy, which is not fully relaxing).

Unwinding reactions experienced include involuntary, spontaneous movements and vibrations, tilting and twisting postures, body sensations, mental images, etc. They are observed with detachment, without participation, and as phenomena that accompanies the flushing out of tension forces to repair the body. The orientation is to be open and aware and to simply recognize all that is experienced, and to let go.

The observer does not participate in the mind's contents but disengages from it and remains constantly alert. Awareness in the abdominal region ensures that all dissolved and diluted forces are flushed downwards, the direction that will clear out tension forces satisfactorily. Awareness gradually dissolves and loosens up the tension in the abdomen to hip region, which in turn causes a releasing effect in all other parts of the body.

By letting go of the forces trapped within and around, practitioners actually enhance the natural exchange of their debased energy with the cosmic, which is the purest form of energy. Supreme letting go produces total relaxation. In total relaxation, the intent is to go deep within to flush out the tension forces, thoroughly and completely. It is a mentally effortless method using understanding and the minimum of mental energy to cultivate subtle radiant 'psychic' energy, the energy of pure vibrations.

The path of Buddhist cultivation of perfect enlightenment is through:

    1. Precepts (rules to uphold multiple, virtuous conduct);
    2. Stillness (of the mind/heart); and
    3. Wisdom (Prajna in Sanskrit)

In the CFQ purification method a "mantra" is used to access and use cosmic energy. The CFQ mantra replaces the precepts and works on the very thing that created the need for precepts, i.e., karma. CFQ meditation is aimed at cultivating Stillness and Wisdom. The CFQ mantra is used to define the psychic energy developed, and its protection from the overwhelming effect of negative forces. Free exchange of energy with the cosmic is facilitated by the practitioner radiating beneficial and loving energies (Sanskrit Metta). The 'loving-kindness' or metta energy generated by the mantra helps to release the radiant Heart energy that neutralizes the attaching effect of dense karmic forces. As the purification or removal is thorough, CFQ is the ultimate relaxation approach capable of karmic cleansing in self-transformation and into cosmic identification with the energy of the finest vibration and the highest quality. Master Yap maintains that the reduction in dense tension or karmic forces brings out the vibrations of the "Pure Heart". Only when the energy becomes purer will the practitioner progress in Stillness of the Heart (which leads to stillness of the body and mind). With nurturance of Stillness of Heart, the egocentric mind is extinguished and 'the One who knows' or the enlightened observer (or bodhisattva in Sanskrit) sees and interprets things as they are (not affected by karma), shifting from an acquired external knowledge to intuitive wisdom called "instinctive knowledge". When ultimate relaxation is achieved, CFQ brings about a joyous state of alertness, free from the bondage of the physical body, and shifts into cosmic consciousness.

Conversations with
Master Yap

Part 1:

After a Melbourne Conference

2

On the Basics of Energy Meditation

Introducing Master Yap

Master Yap, is truly a remarkable healer. Reflecting on his personal life, he told me about his long-standing curiosity about mysticism, the supernatural, and anything that could explain the mysteries of life. He attributed this tendency to having lived from early childhood, in the isolated fringe of a Malaysian jungle terrain where he was born in 1956. Strange phenomena was often experienced surviving this close to nature. This curiosity led, from his teenage years onwards, to ever deeper exposure, intense training, and continual search for teachers and masters of martial arts, meditation, Qigong, yoga, and healing trance states. Some years later, he discovered he could heal others by the simple laying of hands and as the years went by, his confidence in this healing ability grew. He would volunteer to use this ability whenever the opportunity arose and began to develop a certain reputation as a healer.

His formal education, however, was to qualify him as a public accountant by profession followed by setting up his own accounting firm. He would soon marry and raise a family. But he remained dissatisfied with the conventional professional success and social standing and felt unfulfilled. In 1989, at age 32 years, he arrived at a turning point and could not go on without following his heart's yearning which is to help suffering people. Thus he ended his prestigious accounting practice to become a Qigong alternative medicine practitioner, much to the surprise and disappointment of friends and relatives alike.

From the beginning of starting his healing Center in Penang, there never was a shortage of clients. In fact, appointments stretched from early morning to near midnight most days of the week. His unusual healing technique combining the laying of hands, directing energy by pointing his fingers or massaging joints all worked well enough to attract clients, despite much initial doubts.

However, deep within himself the young healer was not impressed with his apparent success. He wanted to understand and learn more to be even more effective. He used energy to heal, and had high expectations of remarkable results that were as yet unattainable but at that time energy healing was largely a mystery. He also had a nagging fear that he was wearing or burning out rapidly. He soon discovered how inadequate he was. So he continued to explore other forms of powerful Qigong healing techniques but much to his disappointment they were not much more effective nor provided the complete explanation that he expected. He was however fully convinced that energy worked, as witnessed by what he saw in his clients. So he kept the faith in pursuing his search.

Then a series of unusual, transforming experiences occurred that he referred to as revelations.*

---

*Master Yap's three-phased initiations (Night of the Hexagram, Goldbody Luminous State, and Golden Light Bodhisattva) that led to the revelations on CFQ are vividly described in the author's, "Tao of Goldbody Energy Healing."

Intuitive wisdom illuminated the principles of energy healing and the answers that fully explained how energy healing worked. He had simply to go into meditation to harness Heart energy that produced the most remarkable cures. At age 35 years, he had finally reached his destined vocation to become a universal healer.

The principles unveiled became the foundations of what Master Yap teaches that he calls "CFQ" (Chaoyi Fanhuan Qigong). It is a direct understanding of how energy transforms the body and frees the spirit toward enlightenment.

CFQ Energy Works

On my return from Australia to Japan, I made a stopover in Malaysia to visit Master Yap,"In Melbourne, I conducted a workshop on Eastern and Western approaches on relaxation and health. How is CFQ energy healing related to Eastern practices such as Qigong?"

CFQ adheres to four Taoist principles universally accepted in Qigong practice. The four sequential steps are: Nourish the essence to convert to qi; Refine qi to convert into Spirit; Refine the Spirit to return to Emptiness, and Refine Emptiness to return to Tao.

Traditional Qigong interpreted these principles as the four processes in practice treating them as four different stages of attainment. One must first learn how to nourish one's essence to turn into qi energy, and then gradually proceed step by step, to each of the other stages in turn.

However, in CFQ practice, all four processes are adhered to, but they are not considered as separate steps, or stages of progressive cultivation. Instead, all four practices are incorporated and done simultaneously in CFQ. Consider the notion of 'nourishing essence to turn into qi'. In CFQ practice, the body is not permitted to move too much or become over-excited, i.e., the practitioner does not waste essence or energy. Spontaneous movement in CFQ is not wasted energy, but a release of what is stored in the body and causing problems. This is in line with not wasting one's essence as it is naturally converted into the essential body energy."

CFQ practice also pays particular attention to the human spirit. The CFQ mantra is used for this purpose, so that at all times the practitioner is reminded of his or her spiritual existence by virtue of the Mantra. The cultivator makes sure that the Mantra is continuously recited. That means the spirit is quite alert, and that it exists all the time. The practitioner does not doze off during practice. That is cultivation in converting the qi into spirit.

"How does CFQ refine the spirit to convert into Emptiness and return to the Tao?"

At all times our consciousness is fully alert. The spirit is purified by means of what we do with relaxation energy. This energy generated during CFQ dissolves the karmic forces from the body, which are accumulated in the form of tension forces. The energy of relaxation is radiant by nature, i.e., it radiates or opens out, and goes back to the cosmos or the Tao. In other words, we empty ourselves of impurities and defilements, to eventually become part of the cosmic conscious-ness. If successful, we return to and become one with the Tao.

In CFQ meditation, all four principles are not distinguished, but practiced simultaneously to attain the goal. Most standard types of Qigong are based on the belief that one had to go step by step, stage by stage as a gradual process. But this is not the right way. When practiced separately to master each step before proceeding to the next, there is confusion and contradiction. In the first two processes, there is a kind of gap between qi and spirit, and confusion of where spirit is to be found. Normally, for example, Qigong say bring the qi up from the lower abdomen to the heart, then from heart to brain, and that is then called spirit. That assumes spirit accumulates in the head. Then one is suppose to return spirit to Emptiness. But CFQ questions whether this is the correct process of the return to Emptiness.

"What then is the correct procedure?"

It must involve a downward releasing. The big problem is that if one already has absorbed and accumulated so much, can one actually want to, or be able to, release anything at all? Then from Emptiness, one is supposed to merge with the path or Tao. My experience is that one step does not lead to another. But, if we practice all four togeth-er, they simply merge together beautifully.

Also from the letting go aspect of CFQ, by trying to keep following complicated processes or systems, that defeats and contradicts the process of letting go. That is creating something, not letting go. That's acquisition, and when one acquires so much, I doubt if one can ever return to Emptiness.

"How is your energy healing system related to meditation with a Buddhist orientation?"

The concept of Tao is the same as the Buddhist understanding of Enlightenment. Traditional definitions of qi refer to it as a very basic force that enables life to function. But qi is defined with different words depending on the type and location in the body. Universal external energy is called "wai qi," and what is in the body is called "nei qi". The Chinese also believe that qi can be absorbed to strengthen the body. This notion, CFQ rejects—one gets healthy by not absorbing, but by releasing. In CFQ, we really do not talk of such ordinary qi energy at all.

CFQ energy healing blends Buddhist meditation with Qigong. The essence of CFQ is more related to Buddhism. A very basic principle in Buddhist cultivation, such as in Vipassana and Zen meditation, is also letting go. In CFQ, when one lets go, the hindrances and defilements are removed in an optimal way, so that whatever needs to happen in the body will be created. Whatever qi required is already present in the body. We just make sure that in practice, we do not create a hindrance to its flow. This is also consistent with the belief in traditional Chinese medicine that when something unhealthy happens, the qi in the body is blocked.

Another Qigong belief is that one can absorb qi from certain foods, by using certain meditation techniques, and from certain exercises. But at the same time they say that when qi is blocked, one should stimulate it, for example, by means of acupuncture, or one can add and subtract qi by food and herbs. But again such practices are based on acquisition, which from the Buddhist point of letting go can become a hindrance. One ought to just let go, and whatever obstructions there are, will clear off by themselves. We say that in CFQ, we harmonize the qi. What is supposed to happen, let it happen—by letting go. We do not interfere. There is no need to quarrel with what qi means, only that acquisition interferes, and we say the letting go approach is better than acquisition.

"Does Buddhist practice imply the notion of energy?"

Indeed, Buddhism talks about energy all the time. Pure energy is called 'Emptiness' or the 'Void', translated from the Sanskrit word, 'Sunyata'. The sacred texts and the Buddha when referring to mind, or to karma, are really referring to energy. The essence of CFQ is the Heart Sutra that is the core philosophy of CFQ. It describes a state of meditation that prevents and does not allow interference by any or all the five senses. Interpretation by one's five senses form a relationship with the impure energy, creating tension whose products are all illusory. Through meditation, one goes beyond, deeper into the pure energy state, which is called Emptiness in the Heart Sutra. When a person is purified, to that extend, that individual will see the truth of all events happening, and will not be deluded by all the physical events happening. It will also help to dissipate and clear out all the undesirable physical events from happening.

The Heart Sutra is often recommended for people to clear off undesirable problems, create better health, and good karma for themselves. Through the attainment of pure energy, one understands and see that all impurities are only illusions. One finds that in the pure state of the 'Unmoved Heart,' when the Heart is not disturbed, all events cease to create a disturbance for them. One sees things in the right perspective.

Pure Heart precisely means cosmic consciousness or energy. Perfect purity is cosmic energy. In CFQ, we refer to Heart energy, and the pure energy of the heart to mean non-participation. It's the ability not to participate or to exist in the unmoved Heart. Not to participate will release the blockages or obstructions, that are normally created by various life processes hindering the qi flow in the body. At the end of it, we are still working on energy.

The development of intuitive wisdom leads to "instinctive" knowledge. When you move into the wisdom or prajna of the Heart Sutra, pure energy shines, and one just see things for what they are. At this stage, you no longer distinguish between pure and impure. One then can see all—the physical, as well as the non-physical impurities. The unrealized person sees only the physical impurities. Such a person will distinguish between impurity and purity. But once enlightened, things are seen just as they are. In cosmic consciousness, one is so unmoved that nothing changes; there is only timelessness. That's the same as enlightenment.

Energy as Antecedent of Disease

"Is the basic objective in CFQ energy therapy a means of inducing the release of an energy-based tension accumulated in the body?"

In terms of energy, all aspects of a human being, whether physical, mental, or spiritual draw tension forces inwards. The energy condensation taking place is a greedy form of force that is stuck in the body depending on where it's created. Normally they are trapped in the whole body inclusive of the head and brain itself. These forces, as they accumulate and solidify in the body, create physical folds, hardening, and shortening of the body. That is the cause of disease. Letting go of the deep stress from energy condensation is difficult to understand until one practices CFQ and experiences the benefits. Body, mind, and spirit all go along in the same direction affected by energy condensation—so it is with psychological and emotional stress.

"There's bio-psychosocial stress and its link to disease effects as defined in Western psychology that most people are familiar with. But in CFQ energy theory is there much more?"

Of course they overlap. For example, when talking about emotional stress, there are many therapeutic ways to release emotional stress. CFQ also talks about that but does not stop there.

"Therapists help people to let go of that emotional trauma to get some relief. Researchers have shown that release of emotional inhibition is healthy. In relation to letting go process, explain how the mind can prevent disease and rejuvenate the body."

Can we first deal with how the stress accumulated traumatizes the body? Whatever stress has been generated, there is a solidification process from the stress energy forming in the body itself. There is a continuous process of solidifying such stress in the body. Each passing minute more stress is drawn inwards and accumulates in various energy centers in the physique. This dense energy undergoes a change in state that is characteristically in glue-form so that the body gets hardened.

"Slow that down, what does hardening mean in biological terms?"

O.K., for instance if you observe a person in a fit of anger, you'll find that the body has stiffened and hardened. So this is a physical and physiological change. The stress process is the same biological mechanism, especially over the passage of time.

"So hardening is a kind of physiological arousal of the body. But you are implying it goes beyond that?"

In hardening, the muscle tightens up, coils, and shrinks inwards in order to spring into action. If this action is not allowed to happen or the coiled energy is not acted upon, then it has to be absorbed completely. The tension doesn't get released. So there is a pattern from the residual energy. Tension released will have a stretching effect and a return to a biologically relaxed state with a resulting improvement in biological function.

"Is there the same hardening mechanism when cells are damaged by excess sugar metabolism and oxidative damage?"

In this context, I'll throw in the notion that the hardening here is caused by energy condensation to its physical counterpart.

"Before talking further about energy, elaborate at a more material level how cellular damage is linked to disease-related aging."

Ah, the missing gap—how to convey the message that energy causes such physical effects? For those who cultivate an energy health practice such as in CFQ, this is a very natural process. Energy, as it becomes more condensed, becomes physical and is experienced as such. The gap is getting the novice to understand that energy and physical force are totally convertible.

Take the process of eating itself. That of course creates a kind of stress on the body. The need to eat is stress driven—The body sends hungry messages because the body responds to the shortage of food. Signals that food is needed create a tension or stress that causes hunger pangs. If that is not fulfilled, there can be digestive damage over the long term. That's also energy, i.e., the nature of stress is energy.

Stress energy also causes aging. To understand this, first understand stress is, in effect, a force that comes from energy.

"Psychologists understand fostering health in terms of the dynamics of stress removal. So stress can be interpreted in terms of its components, i.e., as a physical or biological force and that is transmitted via an energy process to the body and their resultant stress response and disease effects. Stress management is feasible by prevention or releasing the stress force and energy components."

The energy forces store memories as well. Each force has markers or the imprint of specific information captured or associated with its original creation. Traumatic memories, for example, cling to the person in their energy patterns.

"How does the energy store memories?"

Energy has electro-magnetic properties. Consider the stress energy as analogous to the messages in a recording device. These recorded messages are stored as electronic or magnetic signals in the tape. It can also be retrieved energetically or played back or transformed with a tape player. Similarly, this is compatible to stress created during the life process.

Most important is to understand that stress is internalized as energy and through energy condensation becomes a physical force trapped in the body. The physical aspect of stress is the force or the stimulant that causes the stress. That stimulant depends on how a person interprets or appraise it as stressful. That's the stress response as you would call it.

"O.K., going back to the stress in the cells that cause aging. The solution of course is stress resistance and stress reduction. Then we can ask how to enhance the person's ability on stress reduction as a means to slow down the aging process."

We don't say resist stress but how to subtract stress or reduce it. Again we emphasize that stress is energy in physical manifestation. This stress or energy is being deposited, absorbed and accumulated in the body.

"It is not an easy process to get relief from stress!"

It needs a sophisticated system with a proper understanding of the laws of qi energy to remove the stress and get it released. This force, since is has condensed from energy, stresses the body causing a permanent deformation of the physical form or biological body. We have a energy releasing system that provides a way to dilute this force—this causes an opening effect. Once this force is diluted there will be an outward stretching. It's a loosening effect to reverse illnesses.

Reduction of Tension Energy

"When you say stress reduction and subtraction, one sensible method is obviously letting go. Can you explain how letting go can dilute this force or stress and open it out and release it?"

To talk of resistance creates further stress. The word resistance leads to tensing and fighting back and that is stress itself. Fighting to hold back and not allow the stress to go within is futile—stress is such a natural process created by life. We are all equipped with the natural function of the stress response and any attempt to hold back or resist the process may increase the stress itself. So we can talk about a breakdown point. A person may fight very hard to resist the stress but eventually will fail and that creates real havoc to one's health. Resisting has a limiting effect and in the long run counterproductive.

"I can see that people vary in their ability to release stress naturally. Can this be related to people's resilience?"

People varying in resilience also vary in energy patterns. The more resilient type has energy that seems to be more easily activated. The energy is not as hardened and that energy can be changed or released quite easily. For those whose energy hardens more readily, the person becomes more rigid and will be less resilient.

"How can one help people to be more resilient in overcoming adversity and rebound back to health?"

Your problem will be largely solved if you can zero in on making people understand that the stress itself can be energetically explained. When people do understand this they know that this stress is not something abstract but rather is energy in different stages of condensation and that manifest with different physical properties. Then your subsequent explanation of becoming resilient is easy to grasp.

"What do you mean by the different manifestations?"

Again, basically, stress is energy. Get people to accept that, then they can follow the rest easily. All information is energy manifested. And all stimulation is energy manifested as well. So it is in aging as the waste products of metabolism comes about through the process of creating cellular energy.

"So it has to do with the basic ingredient of all matter?"

All physical matter is comprised of energy patterns. All elements of atoms are also energy. So in that manner when we talk about blood glucose or sugar or any nutrient—that is energy is its different forms or manifestation.

"Yes, of course, right. The scientific theory is that aging is the result of cell metabolism slowing down as cells age and as waste by-products builds up."

One source of aging is from the accumulation of sugar. Another source is from oxygen. A third is the hardening of the energy. But in all cases, we are basically referring to energy in different forms. They all translate into energy eventually.

"I see what you mean that it's all energy in its different manifestation whether it's food, or oxidation, or excess sugar glycosylation waste products gluing up cells. These are forms of biological stress. And in addition there's the psychosocial stressors of living. So when letting go of stress, we eventually have to deal with letting go of condensed energy?"

Yes, that also means that stress reduction through drugs will have very limited effect in melting this dense energy off. Drugs can at best carry off perhaps the sugar. But the drug itself leaves behind some by-product with problematic side effects. If the drug is powerful enough to dilute by reacting chemically with the stress agent that will also leave some possibly harmful residue.

"Researchers appreciate that stress can be removed by emotional expression or through social support, or by means of some stress management technique. They lead to the letting go experience of emotional release."

Yes, but you have a partial experience only.

"What is full?"

Letting go is much more than emotional expression as established in conventional psychology. The problem is only partially resolved through releasing it this way since this relief is not total. If you want to be thorough you have got to bring in the life energy concept and the qualitative differences between impure and pure energy. Universal life force is the energy that animates life. When we examine life itself there is a non-physical or unseen force.

For an audience who is more physically-oriented, we would not go much further. But we can say briefly that there is something deeper and what that is. When we refer to science, it does not deal with living energy itself. But to understand life we can't totally avoid touching on the life force.

The Process of Tension Release

"The relaxation effects of meditation and the psychological value of EEG-brain states such as the transcendent-state consciousness are well documented. In the field of transpersonal psychology, the endeavor is to go beyond the personality to an underlying conception of the human spirit. What is the goal of energy meditation in CFQ?"

The system is a means to release the pent-up energy and the unwinding effects during the complete letting go experience that manifests as spontaneous movements. During energy meditation, spontaneous movement itself is evidence that energy itself is actually very physical. That's why there are physical movements. This condensed energy is a form of stress that pulls and shortens the muscles and is stored and accumulated in the physical organs and in the muscles. It has force and direction. If it is released properly it goes out in that way.

It also has memory as I mentioned before. For example, if the movement is in the form of dance where does the dance come from? It comes from a memory associated with the energy or from the imagination of the person. There is information in the memory. So the goal of energy meditation is to release all accumulated stress provoking memories and tensions stored in the mind and body.

"Sounds confusing."

A basic aspect of energy relaxation is spontaneous movement which is a manifestation of the tension energy moving out.

"Is it also the way of letting go?"

It is true that movements are quite a necessary process of energy meditation. But that's not the essence of the way. Some people get this very wrong. It's not the intention to move into spontaneous movements—that will lead to acquiring more stress. I'm referring particularly to trance and hypnosis. Even most types of Qigong techniques that teach spontaneous movements move because of the motive, 'I want more qi power.' Here people will also be moving spontaneously. But in such situations, the conscious mind is shielded off and they are spontaneously moving according to the suggestion. That itself is a strong stress formation.

"How does one differentiate between these two? You say—don't suggest to yourself to move but also assert that in CFQ energy meditation, unwinding has to do with the movements."

In CFQ practice the person has very clear consciousness and that is maintained throughout. Whereas in the hypnotic or trance state, the mind can be quite confused in consciousness. At best they are in a dreamy state and they are very disorientated.

"You are saying that spontaneous movement is not the goal but is one of the processes. The person may not necessarily be doing spontaneous movements when letting go?"

That happens sometimes as there are different things going on during the unwinding process.

Pure Qi-Energy as Tension Solvent

"What other possibilities or processes are experienced in letting go—with spontaneous movements being just one?"

In terms of quality of qi energy the highest grade itself is pure energy. Only when pure energy is brought through properly can it enhance the melting off of stress. That is because of the density of impure energy. By nature, these energies cling and attach themselves to the body. We have to make sure we bring through energy of the right kind or pure energy that is non-attaching and radiates to flush out the dense energies.

"So in CFQ, good energy is used. And this is related to the letting go intention?"

The more impure the energy the heavier it is. That means there's more stress. As you go up the scale in purer energy it is finer in vibration. The purest form of energy is the finest in vibration that is needed in order to melt off the very coarse energy of stress.

"So you are implying two things—The first is that letting go is the intention. Second, that intention of letting go can be facilitated by bringing in pure energy?"

Let me straighten this out. To de-stress is dependent on letting go. The criteria of letting go is that you must make use of good energy. To do otherwise you may not be successful. Let's say the person has the intention to let go. If he does not know how to bring through good energy, conceptually, he will be driving himself to let go repeatedly. He may be driving himself into depression instead of letting go. In that way it is self-defeating.

"The proper way of letting go is dependent on bringing through good energy of the right type. But if one just focus on letting go by itself that can create problems?"

Yes. It leads to depression. It makes a person feel, 'Oh, life is so meaningless.'

"Yes, disappointments in life have a way of piling up. Life is too often full of suffering. So instead of feeling that life is such a drag you have to replace that with a more positive thought?"

Correct.

"So the finest energy can act as a tension energy solvent. That's the Mantra or one's innermost intention you recite silently during energy meditation. The Mantra signifies the thought of pure energy?"

Correct. Basically everything boils down to thoughts and emotions.

"Good or pure thoughts and emotions in relation to the Mantra?"

Oh yes, yes. But again we have to make sure that we know the laws of energy meditation. There should be only minimal thinking during meditation and so the mind process of bringing through the good energy must not be too active. It must be such a mechanical and natural process that hardly any effort is involved in doing so. That ensures the good energy does not become attaching. Once it becomes attached that develops into another form of stress and it doesn't cancel off the previous stress created.

"A central point in energy meditation is the mind focused on good energy that you call Metta, a Sanskrit word that means compassion or loving-kindness. There is, of course, still some attachment while one is bringing in that energy?"

Yes, very minimum. It's so light and so fine. But that is necessary otherwise you will not be able to bring through the energy at all. In order to generate the good energy for the pure cosmic energy to come through, we make sure that the effort used is as minimal as possible.

"Picking a good mantra to focus on may not be easy. You said that focusing on the thought of, 'Let it go!' is not a good mantra because it creates a kind of depression. Then you suggested using the word, 'Good' or its equivalent. But that word is too commonplace and used in too many different contexts and is too misleading. How about the word 'Metta'?"

Of course Metta is a good idea but how many people do understand what Metta is?

"That may be asking too much."

The intent is—Pure & Good! Or better, ask them to device their own mantra according to their beliefs. Give them a strong hint and let them come up with whatever they imagine.

"Pure Perfection sounds good. Or in Sanskrit writing, I think of 'Prajna Paramita' meaning the Perfection of Wisdom."

Yes. But in practice, whatever one's mantra, use it as mechanically as possible so that there is no active thinking involved. We certainly don't want to add more burden by more stressful thinking. Because as you go on in meditation, we are talking about something that is very spiritual or what's deeper than mind. A lot of hardship is involved in developing that potential.

The realm of the human spirit or life energy, however, may be possibly beyond the reach of physical science. For example, you may not be able to measure pure energy because scientific instruments measure entities within a certain degree of vibration. When things are so fine and non-physical, you can't measure that at all. But that does not mean that it doesn't exist.

The Energy of Non-Attachment

"Coming back to a more basic point. The mantra is based on the idea that good thoughts will create good energy. How can this be explained?"

Let's say a person is involved in some good activity by normal standards. The person does something that he or she feels good about and will be happy. That individual's emotional well being is better off in the normal sense, right? Doing something good, the person feels happier emotionally. However, in this instance, the person is doing something good but is attached to the outcome. So the action is still quite coarse in relation to the pure energy. Anything that is purer in terms of goodness is beyond one's conjecture or imagination. We just leave it as a mechanical process for the energy to sort it out. So purity is defined as being non-attaching.

For it to be non-attaching, it is not confined to the normal standard of good. It's beyond that and that means it's a more extended view of one's identity. In other words, there must be a trust involved. It's understood as such.

"Can these ideas lead to new productive ways of dealing with health problems?"

We are moving along the line of purity beyond the normal standard of purity that have yet to be measured.

"But can someone progress with such beliefs?"

That requires you to be involved in it. It goes back to the tradition that such meditative experience is not easy to gain since it's beyond normal expression.

"But can the ideas we've talked about be applied to improve working on an aging disease such as Alzheimer with dementia or AD patients?"

Not an easy process. But in terms of activities, the therapeutic aspect is to cheer them up, provide them games to interest them for them to feel better. That's probably all the therapists can do right now since there's no hope of cure of course. So we congratulate them for doing the right thing. Beyond that they must get themselves right into CFQ training in order to help patients further. That would need a very advanced meditator to do so. Although this is difficult, it must begin with healers knowing about letting go and the meditation potential. They have to break their own barrier of transmitting good energy. At this point, the therapist can only do or help based on the normal standard of goodness.

"What are the conceptual principles involved that others can understand in terms of treatment?"

The tools that I use are derived from my systematic meditation over many years. These are my tools which are not visible. I can bring through the good energy through long meditative experience. Good energy means energy of the finest type that acts like a solvent that can dilute the stress of negative energy that cause AD.

But CFQ can bring it through and cause changes to the patient. A meditator or a healer has got to bring in the right energy that continuously goes through the patient and melt away and dilute the stress. So as you go in you penetrate the layers after layers of stress. The body is full of millions of energy folds that protrude well beyond the physical form. The extent the healer can penetrate depends on how advance the cultivation is. In other words, how much he has dealt with such energy within oneself.

"Medical people will say its not possible to do much since brain scans in AD patients show that the brain is already shrunken."

Very good, but why has the brain shrunk? The answer is that the brain has for long been squeezed by the tension force. The whole body is shrinking as a person ages. It depends on the stress formation within the body. The natural process of aging has, I believe, a shrinking effect on the brain and the entire body. An aging person may have shrunk a few inches from head to toe.

"Yes, that is readily observable in the elderly."

In our experience we have seen how the patient's body can be straightened. As the whole body is stretched, some have gained some height that is measurable over a period of time. In our treatment others who are interested can monitor changes in vital signs such as heart rate, blood pressure, and electroencephalogram or brain wave functions.

"Maybe its time to do some research on this?"

Given the right opportunity—yes. I am confident multiple physiological changes are detectable immediately during treatment. At some point, however, researchers have to understand that they are dealing with the energy or spiritual effect. But energy is also physical.

"Stale energy condenses in the entire body and mind to become a noxious agent that cause disease. To be healed, the trapped energy must be released?"

The healer must be prepared to move into it. All existing treatment is inadequate because it focuses on the body using physical interventions. But we are talking about life. Even traditional Oriental medicine with yin and yang theory have not deviated much from the body itself. This is like forcefully altering or repairing a house without the owner's consent and stuffing the house with toxic building materials. The result is disastrous.

The CFQ viewpoint says that health practitioners need to go all the way into life itself rather than just the body. It is to free noxious agents from one's home and teach the occupant how to maintain it.

Of course, physical intervention like medication is necessary to help people manage their problems when they are already down. But this, at its best, brings only relief. A profound cure can only come from working with the energy or spirit. For anyone with problems, it will not be wise to excessively pursue relief in the hope for a cure as this may cause rapid worsening of the problem. Help-seeking attempts that provide relief when properly used in the right amount can help a person manage the problem and slow down deterioration. Cure comes from working in the opposite direction!

Part 2:

After a Tokyo Conference

3

On Reversing Disease and Aging

In Tokyo, I had presented a symposium on healthy aging. I flew to Penang and met Master Yap or Sifu for the second time. "Sifu, let's begin with the good news about longevity. Human life spans in the developed world continue to increase over the century leading gerontologists to suggest that the human biological time clock can be reset. With longevity increased, healthy aging needs to be promoted to halt the normal progression of illnesses and diseases in the aging process. Practices to prevent predictable age-related illnesses need to be developed. Can you help people to understand your Qi-energy perspective on health, disease prevention and cure?"

Yes, scientific knowledge can stretch life. But in the past, a shorter life span was due to contagious and infectious diseases. In past times in society those who lived to 100 lived a simple life style and were healthy without scientific medical help. Indeed, genes wear out and cell division slows and physical deterioration occurs in living and during aging. We say, 'Dilute and dissolve the dense energy forces' and genes won't wear out.

"Presumably, resilient people have resilient genes so that their bodies can self-repair more efficiently. Human resilience enhancement should be possible by means of activating the cell repair response."

Present attempts to boost genes and DNA using drug therapies may be impossible to stop aging. Drugs can only act at the physical level while what is needed to do the healing work that rejuvenates the body is much deeper—it is in the life force or energy itself. There is a need to talk about the human spirit and know what that means— going beyond acquisition of knowledge and scholarly knowing.

"I am convinced that a transformation of mental and physical self is needed beginning with shifting to a transcendent state. Can you relate this type of information to CFQ?"

To be optimally healthy the physical material world have to be given up to some degree or there needs be a toning down of one's obsessions—ambitions, enjoyment, quest for knowledge, etc. The necessity is to simplify living to understand and know spirit. Two groups will pay attention to this—those who are afraid to die and the elderly. Also, certain younger people also facing non-fulfillment in a materialistic society. These people are born of affluence and have discovered that life is not meaningful enough.

I have read of spiritual teachers teaching people contemplation to balance their minds filled with negative thoughts. But it's impossible as the adult person keeps doing too much that's negative. This way may not work with most people with their accumulated tensions in full swing. Their heavy tension energy need to be directly cleared off. We need a direct method to cut through the glue-like condensed energy that has literally to be torn and broken off from the physical body. The use of fresh energy is needed to harness this process. The average adult in society today has much difficulties to face and a lot to let go. These are all very physical.

"The issues of balance, letting go, and trusting in change are very much the tenets of a Taoist philosophy. Is that also the case in Qigong?"

Whether Eastern wisdom or Buddhist philosophy, the basic notions of how to live in harmony within and without are the same. Qigong is a more practical development originating from Taoism/Buddhist medical and martial arts concepts and philosophy on how to put them into practice. The ancient sage, Lao Tze, was the founder of Taoism but Qigong probably existed before his time.

"Is it true that in Lao Tze's tiny book of wisdom Tao Te Ching, every line is a code of practice?"

Yes, each verse is literally a code of ethics. In other words, Qigong and CFQ principles are in there—the whole idea is to tell you to relax, not to have cravings for things, cravings for experiences. Relax means try not to think, read, work too much to stress and harden the body. You can see that such advice is not very appealing to most people. So we have to compromise in order not to drive people away—accept average enjoyment so that people don't feel too deprived.

"In my experience, CFQ meditation helps me to think better. I attain clearer thinking by alternating between letting go and waiting for creative thoughts."

Practicing letting go you don't deny yourself benefits. The mind is sharper because by letting go your mind is not so clouded by preconceived ideas. So vibrations and thinking become sharper.

"I am able to focus on what's right. Letting go, I have a continuous fresh flow of thoughts. Without letting go, my thoughts seem to stagnate. Becoming more open, I don't seem to get a heavy head."

That's precisely what letting go is all about—you go in and radiate out to dissolve the tensions created from past experiences. Once these tensions are dissolved you're more open to new ideas—They just flow through. This is not in conflict with letting go as life has to carry on. You are still not blindly pursuing material enjoyments, etc.

Roots of Disease

"I spoke to a Japanese professor in Hiroshima doing Alzheimer disease research. It seems the more education a person has, the less likely the disease strikes. The suggestion is that apparently the lowly-educated person is not using the brain as much. One conclusion is that the more you exercise the brain, the less there is of AD. Isn't this inconsistent with CFQ?"

Normally people need sufficient stimulation or they get bored and easily fall victim to AD. Especially with aging and retirement—the person is at a loss because they feel they have nothing to do. But yet active people like former President Reagan is also a victim of AD. In the case of the lowly educated, the depression from a sense of inferiority and the anger from feeling left out from mainstream society are the causes of AD.

"Why is this so?"

When a person is too active or overwhelmed by too much activity, they bother the person too much. Energetically, the tension glues and shuts off the system because one is too involved in it. Up to a certain point, inactivity is good. Beyond that it bothers too much for most people and there is an increase probability of AD. In energy terms as one ages our energy rises, and the body becomes more and more folded. The physical self hardens and shortens with the body becoming folded physically.

Mentally, there's the formation of a sticky oil or fuel all around us and particularly in the head region. For the elderly, the lower limbs also deteriorate and they have great difficulty in walking, lacking control of their limbs. As the energy rises, the lower body is given up—resulting in difficulty in ordinary functions such as walking and constipation.

"Why?"

Functionally, the body is more suspended. There is a lack of ability for energy to reach the lower body starting from the legs. That's because the energy is coagulated in the upper section. I mean, the lower section has hardened without much functional ability. Blood circulation is effected and does not flow vigorously in the lower body.

What is left eventually is a very slow-moving sticky force in the upper portion. The person reacts mechanically and does not have enough mental activity and can work only on the mechanical life functions which becomes more pronounced. Any response beyond that such as new information fails to be assimilated. There is memory loss and anything new is readily forgotten. More recent actions cannot be absorbed or the affected person seems unable to compute any new information.

"So the tensions accumulated giving rise to sticky energy formation blocks off normal perception of the environment?"

From an energy perception, even young people have, in their brain area, a viscous fluid-like substance which as it thickens blocks one's consciousness so that the person needs to sleep. Sleep allows the body to sort out stimulations to be assimilated and stored in the body. As this process is completed, the person wakes up from sleep. That's the normal sleep cycle.

As a person ages, this force becomes thicker and thicker and energetically can be seen as a dark cloud. It is not only within the body but beyond physical boundaries—everywhere. They are more pronounced in the whole head, including the eyes, nose and ears. That's why the five senses become more impaired over time culminating in old age diseases like cataracts, loss of smell, and lost of hearing. This viscous fuel or force is actually within the body's physical tissue and around it. As it expands out from the body, it is seen as a huge cloud. It feels to the meditator like a mountain. It is hard to penetrate through—it's very bouncy.

Only after years of continuous practice, will it eventually thin out. The thinning-out process feels very physical. In CFQ practice, this force or energy is brought down always starting from the abdomen. As this hard stuff gradually becomes loosen, it goes out from the body gradually which also becomes loosened. The loosening effect goes up to the head.

"So how does the lower body become diseased first?"

That is often the case—a diabetic person is concern about his legs—there is higher risk of amputation. An older person has difficulty walking and needs a stick. Often, older people walk with heels barely touching the ground—That's the suspending effect. Logically in the elderly's weak condition, the feet should be firmly grounded but instead he or she walks on tip-toe. The person walks as if hanging or suspended. Energetically, the psychic heart, which is located near the physical heart, is the location where all forces are linked. We can say that it is one of the most abused spots in the body.

Type II diabetes develops later in life via unhealthy lifestyle such as diet or lack of exercise. But if one is prepared to change and take care of oneself, there's better control of blood sugar. For those less serious cases, such diabetics may get well. The immediate cause of the problem is worked on and then repaired. Whereas for Type I, medicine thinks it's not possible because it's linked to genetics—there is no obvious known cause for the pancreas malfunctioning. In Down's syndrome—Jack's case in Fredericton, the Type I diabetes changed with surprising results when worked on. CFQ works on the spirit and this can literally change the genetic composition.

"True, but Sifu you were not there long enough to cure it."

I have treated other cases in Penang with incurable Down's syndrome effectively. Type I diabetes have been fixed too. There's a nine year old boy that I am currently working on. After one year of CFQ treatment, he is going to school as normal which he couldn't do before. When he first came, he could walk but stumbled badly. Now his physical appearance has changed dramatically—originally he had a very elongated head pointed toward the back. Now the head is rounder and less deformed. His walking is much better.

Another case is a four-month old infant born with a very deformed face—obvious Down's syndrome. She couldn't move her head and her whole body was very thin. She also had congenital heart disease. After the first session, that very night, suddenly she was kicking in the bed. Her grandmother lifted her up and she was able to push herself up and hold up her head. She had the strength to support herself. After the second session of treatment, I warned the mother that the tensions were being flushed out and there may be fever in the child. The child went home and developed a fever but the mother became so frightened she dared not come again!

"Sounds like you're insisting that CFQ can even influence the genes?"

Yes, I am positive.

"How does that work?"

Genetic makeup is a physical expression of innate tension pattern that is physically manifested. CFQ, working as anti-tension agent, clears off the tension, diluting it, so that genetic imbalances or imperfections can be corrected. When the tensions are opened out, the genes change. Environmental manipulation of this sort can change the genes without using drugs.

"So you're saying that the mind can have that influence?"

Mind when expanded deeper goes beyond as the human spirit which is the life force itself. It's not the 'hardware mind' here. Our meditation system works on the life force itself and hardly has any limits in benefits.

"Scientists now can double and triple the lifespan of invertebrates. Through selective breeding—say using worms by stressing them such as raising their temperature by one degree—some worms die. But the hardy ones survive and they now live longer and healthier."

All life forms are sensitive to their environment or surroundings. As a kid, a hobby was breeding tropical fish—swordtails in an aquarium. One can induce color change in pregnant fish by roughly shaking them to excite the fish. After that, the fry grows with new colors such as red eyes.

"Physical stress result in DNA mutations. This suggests that in life span extension, the biological time clock of simple animals, in terms of aging, can be reset. They become stress-resistant living longer and healthier."

Of course for humans too, those who are stress resistant are the ones alive today as those with less stress resistance would have died out.

"Such research led to identification of certain genes which became activated and damage from the stress can be repaired by these special genes. Other research to prolong life is feasible through caloric restriction or starvation in monkeys."

Yes, one traditional belief is that a person who eats less lives healthier and longer.

"The starved monkey was slower to mature sexually, smaller in size but had lower blood pressure, and low cholesterol, i.e., healthy. The researchers expect the monkeys will live longer. Apparently, with slower growth and lengthened developmental phases, life can also be stretched longer."

Yes, I tell my students to eat less and live healthier. The animal instinct is to eat extra to build up reserve for future needs. Today, for humans with food in abundance, this instinct goes on at great intensity—people continue to eat and crave for more. Overeating itself will feed the tension and someone down with nervousness or anxiety will feel induced to continue to consume even further. For these people, with overeating comes the desire that they are not eating enough and desire to consume food supplements.

"Westerners appear to age faster than people here because of high-fat, high-protein eating. They develop much faster, mature sexually earlier, and in the life cycle changes, aging may occur sooner. There is a big gender difference in longevity—women and grandmothers live longer than males because of evolution. They bear and nurture children so their role must in Nature's eyes be more important than men's. Hence women live longer—they have greater value."

In CFQ we go back to basics—often they are forgotten. When practitioners divert from them we pull them back to the basics.

"Why is diversity in activities healthy and even protects the brain?"

People who don't follow CFQ practice need stimulation to go on pro-vided these are not overwhelming. Otherwise they will be knocked down. With CFQ and learning to let go, one realizes that such excita-tion is not necessary to carry on life. We don't need a 'go-go' stress-provoking attitude on an everyday basis to survive. We need only to let go.

"Apparently, people don't understand balance here. Because brain activity is found to be good, people assume that the more the better to improve memory even further. But they forget the possibility of overload. This is the same with exercise—if a little is good, than the maximum must be optimum. And the same with alcohol, nutrition etc. We know that more becomes less where damage exceeds bene-fits."

"Again health research has established that connecting with oth-ers, or having social ties is extremely important but balance is also needed. Take socially-insulated cultures such as Indian tribes living far from others. Surprisingly, their blood pressure remains constant with age throughout their adult life unlike urban cultures. When this was initially discovered, the incorrect conclusion was that they must have a healthier diet. Later we found that once these people living simple lifestyles moved into urban society, their blood pressure go up like the average person in modern societies even though they retain their diets. Now there's a different conclusion about their blood pres-sure—the cause is attributed to their living in socially-insulated cul-tures away from the noise, the bustle and stress of modern societies. So rising blood pressure is not due to biological causes but the result of normal or ordinary stressful living."

"We need some amount of most things in life—exercise, food, activ-ity, friends, etc. But often one gets carried away with wanting more and more and soon forget that you need some peace for your own self. So that suggests to me that, on a daily basis, some time set aside for social isolation is beneficial away from friends and social stress."

That's a good time to practice CFQ.

The Cancer Debacle

"I have witnessed you performing some near miraculous cures on advanced cancer patients that their doctors have given no hope of surviving. Can you present your views about why cancer is so difficult to treat?"

Let me explain by elaborating on what cancer is from the CFQ perspective. Then we can go into what causes prostate problems as well. A body that becomes tensed ultimately produces sticky, folded cells and is 'deformed' physically hindering circulation. We know that everyday the body needs to remove a tremendous amount of toxins and dying cells need to be replaced by new ones. These products have to be removed by the body. But it's life itself that creates the tension that is stored and becomes hardened, enfolding the body into deformations.

This can hinder or obstruct the removal or natural regeneration process. It may trap some of the waste that have to be removed and are not properly released. If these wastes stay on too long it starts the body decay. Decay is acidic or corrosive. Once decay sets in, it eats into the healthier cells. These decaying cells will refuse to die and struggle to survive. But that struggle makes them deformed, mutating with multiple nuclei.

The cancerous cells actually become decay-resistant cells. While resistant to decay they serve their function to hold or check the decay. These cells form into a lump or a tumor. But if this decay is checked, then there's no danger of it spreading further. You're safe—everyone has such pre-cancerous cells to a different degree. Everyone probably has cancer cells but most are not detected. But as more tension accumulates, more decay will continue to set in and as conditions for the process increases, the decayed cells seep through and the cancer spreads causing more cells to become decayed.

"Sorry, what does decay mean biologically?"

It's a kind of corrosion because the dead cell toxins have not been properly removed. It becomes acidic and eats into the body. So it's toxic waste that destroys healthy cells. But these healthy cells will fight back and become deformed in the process and that is cancerous cells turning into tumors. If this toxicity seeps in further, the cancer spreads because more deformed cells develop to wall off the decay.

Usually, the immune system will destroy cancer cells. That is, provided that the toxic materials causing decay have been taken out. As the decay factor moves on into the major blood vessels, the decay may be removed. Then the cancer cells will die off automatically because now there is no more corrosion. No more decay. Then the cancer cells will die off and become replaced by a new generation of normal cells.

"Researchers tell us that cancer cells are a type of cells that are immortal—they multiply endlessly. Most other cells have a division limit before they decay."

Cancer cells appear strongest but they are also the weakest. They are strong because they stubbornly resist adverse conditions, the conditions of decay—if they survive the decay practically nothing can destroy them. But they are also the weakest, because once the factor of decay is removed, they die off rapidly and the body repairs itself.

"How?"

Because they live on the decay itself—parasitically they live on the toxic wastes. They are decay-resistant. You mention earlier about the value of early detection in cancer prevention. However, if the decay cannot be checked or stopped that means it is already spreading and will continue to spread. But the other form of decay that has already been checked will now be static meaning that it won't be diagnosable.

There are two notions—one is that malignant cells will keep spreading. Conventional medical treatment works on the cancer cells or on the parasitic decay in the cells. But unfortunately, these decay cells have roots. If you cut the top off, the roots will continue to grow as a new 'rubbish dump' is created. If you surgically operate and cut it off, the roots will survive independently and spread elsewhere. The parasites need a new rubbish dump.

"I read there's research on a new treatment for cancer, where instead of trying to destroy cells directly, they starved off the cells by weakening or eliminating the blood supply to them. The healthy cells are not effected."

Yes, but it's still very much at the experimental stage. Whether this will pan out is still unknown. It may be as effective as present radiation treatment. Although based on a different strategy the assumption remains the same that cancer cells are the perpetrator. But I say no, the cancer cells are the victims!

The cancer cells are trying to help the person survive the decay. That's why they become cancerous. Otherwise, instead of the containment, the body will have become extensively corroded. That means everything will be destroyed. That happens when the cancer cannot be controlled. The flesh will actually drop off and the bones can be visible. In some of my cancer patients that's exactly what I see.

"I hear that some patients have a rotting smell around them?"

Yes, because of the decay, toward the very terminal stage. When this becomes so apparent there's nothing to control it. It's finally hopeless because the decay rate accelerates too fast.

"I haven't heard this explanation of cancer."

That's right in our CFQ principles. The condition for the decay to set in or the very cause of it is the tension and life itself is full of it. Every passing day, we are more stressed out, and there's more formation of folds in the body. And this prevents proper circulation. So toxins accumulate and as they accumulate to a certain level and given the right conditions, depending on what is stored in the toxin, it may trigger a decay process. Once that takes hold, it is cancer.

People are, of course, many times more afraid of cancer than many other diseases—the pain, and illness that can wipe out the person literally. That also comes from a phobia instigated by negative conditioning from medical propaganda. There is a continuous monitoring and checkups to detect cancer which may not always be necessary but people are scared. The fear generated comes not only from a medical concern for humanity but the business side of the health care industry. When you put this fear into people, people make poor choices.

In the case of fear generated by medical treatment, we may ask, 'Is it better to know more about it or be ignorant about the information available?' To be sure, such information can be advantageous, but not if it's excessive. My belief is that if medical science cannot treat a certain disease, it creates more harm in constantly reminding the person of the disease. The person becomes fearful of it and fear itself creates a kind of negative energy. That can even click on a self fulfilling prophecy and lead a person to that kind of disease.

"Yes, but the truth is that cancer can be terribly painful to treat in comparison to other diseases the radiation, the nausea, disfigurement and wasting away physically. For cancer, we have to examine carefully the treatment implications. It's common knowledge that many cancer treatments simply don't seem to work. It's also a common belief that treatment provides some benefits to the patient."

But to what extent is this true? For example, a person is encouraged to go for the annual cancer checkup. Say the man goes regularly, and then one day he discovers that he has got a cancer that is at an early stage. He goes for the normal treatment—radiation, chemotherapy, and endures the pain of the treatment. After that, with all the fear and propaganda about cancer, his mind is never rested and at ease again. Living in fear, he has nightmares, he can't sleep properly, and because of the worry and anxiety he is unable to work properly.

Some time later, the cancer reappears—that's usually two years later. Most people will then form the wrong conclusion that luckily these patients had gone for treatment and that's why it became possible for them to live these past two years.

But consider another fellow, a happy-go-lucky type who knows little about cancer in terms of early detection and prevention. He also gets cancer but doesn't go for medical treatment nor does he bother to remind himself about this. Essentially, he forgets or drops the matter. So the situation and cancer continues. For argument's sake, this continues without change for another 10 years. Then one day he finds that he feels really bad. He can't eat, he has all the other symptoms. He goes for a medical checkup and discovers he has cancer and it's already terminal. Now he has at best six months to live.

But now compare the two people above. The latter cancer person lived happily for 10 years until the final stage. He did suffer but only in the last six months compared to the first case. He did not have to bear the pain of treatment itself. So do we congratulate the first person for taking the medical treatment? Of course, in reality, the fellow who did not treat the problem seriously might succumb to cancer within months. In real life it's hard to compare but we usually congratulate ourselves for early diagnosis and get early treatment. My point is that it's not always best to assume that a drastic treatment is better than no treatment. I believe that the alternative scenario is often true. The person who does not bother about whether he or she has cancer may live with it undiagnosed until a ripe old age!

"I can see this is possible for the sake of argument. But take prostate cancer, statistics clearly show that if detected early it is curable. But if detected too late, the cancer cells metastasize and spread to other parts of the body and becomes incurable. While confined only to the prostate gland, surgery and radiation therapy can stop it. This supports the general medical advice to go for regular checkups."

Yes, it's difficult to shake that. But how long does it take for the cancer to spread to other places? 10 years? 20 years? One never knows how long before it spreads. You said the malignant cells can be surgically removed. But consider another factor. Later on, the disease could manifest itself in a different formation and the cause may come from the shock of the surgery on the body. The surgery is tension itself—it hardens, coagulates, and further deforms the person. Of course, it's difficult to prove that the cause can be traced to the surgery itself. But I believe that this adds on further to compound the person's health problem.

"You have used a general word—decay—to describe the cancer including figuratively the smell of death."

Cancer cells are victims that try to but fail to prevent cancer. But going back to cases of people who are able to ignored the fear of cancer as a death sentence and the inevitably of death. Probably much of the cancer in the body would have been in check and that person could live to a full ripe old age without developing or getting into full blown cancer. Fear itself can actually create the right condition for it to speed up its growth and the body's deterioration. Of course, there is a percentage who cannot hide by being ignorant of the problem.

"For someone who practices CFQ and has cancer, what should the attitude be...just ignore these fear propaganda? How does one do that?"

If I know the person, I will talk to, and help the practitioner understand fully and convince him or her not to be worried about the problem and that it will be cleared off in CFQ practice or treatment. Then together with getting rid of the disease causing tension, the cancer can be halted. I still don't think conventional Western medicine has an easy way to treat cancer because if cancer cells are cut off, the roots of decay will find a new rubbish dump and start off from there. Burning it by means of radiotherapy produces more dead cells in the body and that means the body becomes more deformed and even more conducive to decay. The cells that are destroyed still depend on the body to remove them. Otherwise, a series of decay phenomena sets in also.

You trust the body to dispose of the damaged and wasted cells. But the weakened body will be less and less able to do so to remove the dead cells. That's why cancer sets in and with the rapid killing from treatment, the body will be unable to dispose of them. These cells will quickly turn into decayed cells and that is cancer.

One says that the treatment can't control it because the cancer has spread but it is precisely the treatment that cause the new series of cancer to develop. So it's the same with chemotherapy—the poison kills so many cells in the body. Of course in medical jargon, the body supposedly will be able to dispose of the dead cells. On that basis, medical treatment is justified in killing off so many cells. That's really a fat hope, an unrealistic hope indeed. In the first place, if the body is able to dispose of all the dead cells, that will mean cancer will not occur. As a person ages you cannot expect that the person can deal effectively with this disposal either. As more tension accumulates in the body the functional ability of the body is reduced—that includes the removal, from the body, of dead cells, removal of toxins, and the ability to regenerate.

It is very unrealistic to trust that the body can do this effectively after you kill the cells by poisoning them with chemicals. So after chemotherapy the cancer recurs. That could well have come about from the treatment or surgery itself rather than factors independent of the treatment. Well, this is an allegation that can't be proved either way. But from our viewpoint, it's certainly very probable. But we have previously mentioned about successful CFQ treatment of multiple cases just by relaxing the person. Also by being more relaxed, the patient copes better with cancer with the additional help of social support.

Once the patient feels more safe, that itself is one of the best ways to approach cancer. That means the patient doesn't worry about it.

For a terminal patient, it makes a difference if you can help make the person stop worrying about cancer. It makes a difference in prolonging the cancer survivor's life and in reducing suffering from the disease. Certainly for a healthy person it will make even more of a difference to remain healthy.

CFQ can be of tremendous help even in a terminal case. It may not be too late provided there is direct energy transmission and meditation practice combined together. The effect is almost immediate unless the patient is very weak and paralyzed. Or unless chemotherapy had been administered and the patient shows signs of rapid deterioration.

But most patients cannot be expected to trust CFQ fully. Most often, they are, at best, taking it as a supplementary treatment. And one can't say anything negative about conventional medical treatment that they are undergoing nor of the negative implications of such treatment. One cannot talk to them frankly. They get angry with me because I would be accused of spoiling their hopes. And since they are already in medical treatment, we also hope that the patient would have full faith in the treatment—it may reduce the harmful effects and help them to cope better with the cancer.

Although I know that conventional intervention is not the best treatment or the best choice, since the person is determined and chosen this, it's better to encourage the patient than to talk against it. You won't be successful anyway to convince the patient to do otherwise. So if you can't convince the patient then its better to encourage rather than to shatter their hopes.

The cancer patient will be in a state of panic. So it's difficult to know what to say and it depends on the individual's mentality—How open the person is, how receptive or fixed, and whether he or she has made up their mind about treatment. But if the person doesn't accept CFQ wholeheartedly, that treatment will also not work well. Yes, because the cancer cure is a time-consuming process and a tough fight. With full cooperation maybe we can work it through even in the advanced stage.

"Why is cancer so tough compared to other diseases?"

First and foremost, there is so much phobia about it. We are fighting for time to heal. Once it's confirmed that it's spreading that means the cell decay rate is accelerating fast. People then often become so depressed upon hearing the news. Many will stop going to work to seek treatment. This is one of the greatest mistakes made by a person diagnosed with cancer! Such a step gives the patient plenty of time to dwell on negative thoughts which in turn leads to depression which accelerates deterioration.

I strongly recommend that they continue normal work and activities, but of course at an easier pace. And then there are some who frantically swallow every known remedy including so-called secret herbal formulas recommended by friends or the latest fad. This is a big gamble to take—that may be enough to kill even a healthy person.

"But they say that cancer is just the tip of the iceberg, that before cancer occurs many things in the body have shut down."

I fully agree with that. Even with just a small lump on the surface, deep within, a lot is already damaged by the cancer even though medically it still can't be detected. So it's not one system but multiple systems everywhere that are linked together. The cancer is discovered at the superficial level, on the skin or muscle itself. But things very deep inside are also damaged.

For example, breast cancer. A small lump on the breast, if examined energetically, may involve a big chunk of stale energy—a lethargic force or very black cloud that completely fills up the lung, the heart, and the whole of the chest area and perhaps penetrating through the back. The muscles at the back between the shoulder blades are often swollen and sensitive and the upper back muscles appear much thicker. Maybe we can see a sort of energy tentacle seeping into the brain. Yet, the external manifestation is only a small cyst-like growth in the breast. So you have a mastectomy to remove the breast but that may speed up the cancer spreading internally, worsening it.

A person comes to the healer who can sense there's breast cancer. We work on it and sense that a certain energy feature in the breast has deteriorated. We go in and see a large chunk of the deterioration as stale energy tension in the lung and chest area. The decay seems to cut in going up to the nose and to the brain. And of course in the digestive system as well. You can even sense that the person may not live long. But then it is the job of the healer to reverse the process, so we quietly work the problem away without even mentioning that to the patient. To be too candid can materialize another illness and reduce the chances of reversing the problem.

The healer knows there's a problem but the person is still considered as medically healthy. In our assessment you feel something serious that is not quite right. At that point in time, the person may complain of a stiff shoulder. She doesn't know there is something far more serious there. When we work on it, there is a sense of penetrating pain, like a sharp knife that stabs through the breast to the back. That means the breast will feel painful and the pain will shoot into the lungs and through the shoulder blades. But she only feels a deep pain and a big chunk deep inside. Of course we will clear that off and we feel happy for them. We also know that this person may have cancer that have been cleared by us without their knowledge.

As I work on the patient she will experience, as unwinding experiences, all the phenomena that is suffered by a cancer patient although less intense. But she is not aware of that as cancer hasn't been diagnosed yet.

"Why is there more breast cancer in the West?"

Oriental women are slimmer and have less tissue. More tissue means greater scope for tension deformation and cancer development. To put it simply, a large breast is statistically more likely to have breast cancer than a smaller one.

Now regarding your earlier question about prostate cancer. Remember I teach that we must relax the whole body and the stale energy has to go down and out. When doing standing meditation, I ask my student to relax the 'Kuah'. That's a joint in the hamstring close to the hip and there's where tension formation develops as the forces become more suspended. The whole lower abdomen and the hip itself becomes hardened. That's also on the sex organ as well. That's why as a person ages the man is liable to be impotent with erectile problems, or for women, menstrual problems and in time menopause itself.

Entangled in Disease: From A.D. to E.D.

"You have some interesting beliefs about what contributes to another disease of aging—Alzheimer's disease or A.D."

A.D. or dementia in general is comparable to a waking dream state as the energy is dense and lethargic. That means it moves very slowly as the energy keeps rotating and there is a play of images all of its own. The person seems to be cut off from all other faculties and comprehension of the external environment. Even as someone talks to the patient, such a person can only stare blankly. The biological system doesn't seem to compute as the energy is too busy rotating from the lethargic forces—the routine life function that remains and goes on is only mechanical.

"This stupor and incomprehension sounds like the brain isn't functioning properly?"

Yes, the whole head region, upper torso, and even the heart area seem to be blanketed by layers of dense and dark forces that keep spinning in the physical structure of the body as well as all around it. These forces will cut off any new information so that any new input can't get into the system. It's still possible to carry on at a minimally mechanical level and to vocalize during the dream state.

"The A.D. person talks about things that appear completely out of touch with reality. You are saying they are essentially dreams that are occurring in their minds?"

The patient is just vocalizing them, but to another person it doesn't make any sense. You can't change that because you can't wake the person up from that dream. He or she doesn't understand what others are saying.

"But does the patient know what he's saying to himself?"

He may understand as he is directly picking that out from his waking dream and saying it aloud. Word for word, it's from the dream itself. And since he is seeing the information and pictures from the dream, he is trapped in that. Anything happening outside at that point is irrelevant—whether it's people who know him well, their names, etc. At a different point in time, different dreams come in and some are less dense than others. So there may be different degrees of recognition—when it is less dense he seems to recognize something out in reality but if it's very dense he seems totally in his own world.

"Many A.D. people wander out of the homes and don't remember where they are and how to get home."

Sometimes they are O.K. At other times, they temporarily wake out of their dreams. But they easily fall back into them because these forces keep accumulating and become denser as dreaming goes on.

"It seems that many people with A.D. have a lower level of education. Why?"

From the energy perspective, a person with a lower level of education who remains content with that does not have a problem. If such people are satisfied with their status or situation they can certainly live to an old age without A.D. In contrast, a person with a lower education level and a restricted range of activities may live in constant discontent or living all the while in the past. Even in their younger days, they dream of things that they can't achieve. So the constant discontent builds up the tension and they become more and more tense psychologically.

"I suspect that this is also a problem for those at the retirement age or for people who are forced into early retirement."

Right. Having reached the established retirement age, the person is considered unproductive. For those who are then unable or unwilling to find activities to fill up their time sufficiently, they will indulge in idle thoughts and frustrations quickly drifting into dream-like states. This is more appealing than hard reality resulting in rapid deterioration of mental and physical health. Even for those who continue to work, they may be easily frustrated as subconsciously they believe that time is running out for them.

Now for those people with low education but yet are not bothered by it, this simplicity means that they are not carrying a heavy mental load. That means less chances of accumulating tension—Tension accumulates at a slower speed. This depends however, on their level of contentment—with low contentment, this will increase their rate of tension accumulation resulting from this discontentment. And in old age when they go into the dream state they naturally drift into unfulfilled dreams.

"There are differences between senility and A.D."

We focus on their similarity—the dementia component, as mentally they are not there anymore. Each creates different patterns of dementia, but across these patterns there are similarities. Energetically, we examine the general pattern rather than their specific differences.

"A.D. effects about four million Americans and researchers have yet to develop a test to diagnose it early, let alone cure it. But one thing is clear—the damage caused by brain lesions and brain tissue marked by tangled brain cells matted by plaques increase exponentially with age.

"Do you distinguish between specific diseases in terms of different tension patterns?"

Tension accumulation in the body, in terms of energy, is a highly complex accumulation. Our assumption is everyone has many or potentially all types of diseases as the body deteriorates and old age sets in. The individual manifestation of the specific disease depends on how he or she has functioned in the past. But this is a minor influence in comparison to the general structure of it.

"Again, how does the tension patterns vary in different diseases?"

Tension accumulation is extremely complex. Tension, for it to exist, means the physical tissues have hardened. The multiple complex forces come from different directions that coalesce into knots and folds of different composition. I find that for heart disease, for instance, their composition also varies from person to person. We are saying that tension forces accumulating builds up everywhere. This is consistent with forces absorbed into the body that have properties of being inward-drawing and upward-suspending and that creates a complex formation.

"How would you treat A.D.?"

We were talking about waking a person from a dream. You find that the moment you send in the healing energy that dissolves the tension the person feels a sudden loosening—Pop! Like a bubble bursting or a taut string that's cut suddenly. Something pops off from the head and the patient is suddenly awake. But as you work further and penetrate deeper, something else forms into a bubble-like thing or plastic cover that will bind-up the person again. Then the person drifts back into dreaming again. But persist and work longer and the bubble will burst again and the person will be awakened out of it.

So it's very complex and hard to come to a concrete definition and very time consuming. A satisfactory treatment may take a hundred energy healing sessions over a period of two or three years. A major consideration whether to treat an AD patient is whether the person has sufficient opportunities to develop activities to keep fully occupied. It can be hobbies, house-keeping, gardening, even gossiping.

"Actions matter and not thoughts and dreaming."

As the treatment goes on, someone must help the AD patient to be involved in such activities. The person will be cured when fully occupied.

"What about the psychological state of the person?"

It's easier to look at a persons' behavior. For example, a easily-angered person is more likely to suffer from elevated blood pressure, heart disease, and stroke. A chronic depressor who holds on to some kind of secret worry, unable to express hidden fears is more susceptible to cancer. From the energy point of view, any differences between diseases are irrelevant—we have just to work through the different complex layers. When the person is suffering from a heart disease, it is obvious that the area that is totally hardened is in the heart region. It is the middle torso that is totally hardened. But as you work further, you discover that the disease is also in the head, the hip, and even the toes. Everywhere!

Again, it's a waste of time and resources to go into details. The danger is that you may neglect the importance of the overall tensions. For example, for heart disease, you can almost certainly find evidence of heart disease even in the energy in the toes. Heart disease means that it's very dry. It can also be very 'heaty' leading to the eruption of heart disease. As you work beyond it, it becomes cold. The heat is just the surface symptom though. The underlying cause is the same. You release the tension and depending on how much of that is released, the person improves.

"Erectile disease or E.D. is a common affliction."

For men, one problem is prostate enlargement. First, it becomes hardened as the energy or force is so suspended. The tension is everywhere in the hip and in particularly in the sensitive prostate gland and is readily manifest as physical problems.

"What about Viagra?"

It is a drug and so has a stimulating effect. If you have a stressed-out person, a drug can suppress his nervousness by making his mind more lethargic. It seems to solve the anxiety problem. But that of course is not a real solution. Viagra stimulates the body perhaps by stimulating blood flow to the lower body that boosts his confidence. But with CFQ, I can tell you that in a few cases, my students have such a problem. After two to three months of practice it's gone!

CFQ Energy Meditation: The Heart of Metta

"Meditation is an essential tool to cultivate letting go efficiently. But there are many forms that are already available and taught. Meditation is a long, arduous discipline with no guarantee of success."

Yes, meditation! But why and what is meditation? It is a process to discover your true self that one can call the 'God within' or to free the Buddha trapped within you. That is the motivating factor as defined traditionally by Buddhism and Taoism. It is definitely not about attempting to relax physiologically, as true relaxation comes only after one discovers that higher or true self within. It is also absurd to meditate for supernatural powers, cure diseases, acquire and create wealth, or expand one's knowledge. Such seeking is motivated by extreme greed traditionally scoffed at and called, 'Zen of the wild foxes.'

To meditate with the wrong motivation itself brings disastrous effects, although in the short term it appears fulfilling because of the appealing effect of its promises. The right intention is to discover one's true self, and with proper guidance and perseverance, the benefits of relaxation, ridding of diseases, etc., come as fringe benefits.

I agree meditation techniques have to be gradual and few can swim out of quicksand by themselves. Insight meditation can be perfected by monks who trained from childhood practically living all their lives in forests. They probably don't know what social stress is all about really other than conceptually. Any layperson will have tremendous difficulty learning such techniques.

"But if we suggest using more contemporary methods such as CFQ, they feel that since it is so different from their traditions that it must be a watered down diluted version of the real thing. So energy meditation is superficial because it is not following what is prescribed in ancient texts."

We can capture them by pointing to the ultimate goal of Qigong that advocates Stillness—stillness of the heart, stillness of the body, and mind. That will lead not only to perfect health but beyond to ultimate wisdom and enlightenment.

"How does one achieve such an ultimate goal?"

We can equate all the tension energies accumulated in our lifetime in one word—karma, a Sanskrit word which means action, or deed. Karma is basically composed of all of one's past experiences that encompasses one from cradle to death, and perhaps before. One can go back further and further to the infinite past. First, one must be able to cleanse the karma beginning with our most recent tension energy.

"I understand karma is the law of causality. In psychological terms, we become what we think, feel, and behave. What happens to us is the effect of previous actions and the energy carried forward. How does one break that off as an adult already in a state of high stress?"

Indeed one's karma is already in full manifestation. But we say, 'Look we have a technique that can promise ultimate Stillness of the heart, the mind, and the body. From that, one reaches perfect wisdom which is the highest goal.'

"Again how does one attain that?"

We have a technique to cut through the tension karma. Without the ability to cleanse out the karma one will be carried and swept away by the dense energy. All the time, we engage in daily activities that creates karma and without a strong technique to cut through the karma, nothing will work. If the meditator emphasizes too much on artificial Stillness of the body, one is still bounded by the ego asserting itself. This is karma clinging to the ego. First, begin with the Heart. Since the body-mind-spirit are so completely entangled by the karma, we have got to create a new feature here. This new feature is your innermost intention which is a detachment from this karma.

"Why the emphasis on the Heart? I recall Acharn Chah, the great Vipassana or insight meditation teacher and forest monk, saying that the first thing is listening with your Heart!"

What is meditation's goal but to realize your true or real self—Where is your real self? One's real self is the innermost. What is the innermost? That's the Heart. It's in the Spirit—That's where all the karma binds together. The physical body is only like a bag.

When we say the word Heart energy, we mean the innermost energy or innermost intention or desire to purify oneself. Only with such intention can you eventually break away from the bondage of karma itself. Karma defines all your activities and actions and the cause of life itself. Since a person is already bound-up by his or her karma, whatever the individual does or says is defined by such karma.

You have to create a new intention—that is a new series of functional patterns. So detach your Heart from the existing karma. Take it out. Learn how to bring through the right energy because basically karma is energy created that draws the problem into us. You must learn to bring through the right kind of energy. It is Metta or Heart energy which melts away the karma. If given proper merits the karma will eventually melt away. It dissolves and get diluted. Without this Metta element, nothing will work.

In the layperson, it appears the Heart is nowhere to be found. The person is totally bound up by karma from the surface to the deepest interior. The karma defines how an individual looks at the world, where one is going, when one will suffer, and how one is going to die. It determines how the person's appearance changes with age too. And spiritually this bundle is a heavy load on the individual.

Karma, seen psychically, is a black cloud-like formation as information, etc.. A layperson could be said to almost have no Heart, i.e., everything about him is purely defined by the karma. The Heart within the karma is totally hidden. One has to instill a new feature in him.

"Explain what is Metta and where that comes in?"

The intention is towards good—That itself is Metta. Karma is energy with impure identities. They have defining qualities such as heaviness, denseness, and negativity. They are slower in vibrations. The purer the energy goes, the finer it is and the better the quality and the faster the rate of vibration. Metta is pure energy manifested as loving energy or compassion.

One brings in the right kind of good energy that is non-attaching as define by CFQ principles—not narrow but is a non-attaching good. That's the purest form of energy or Metta. If you bring through the purest form of energy, it won't cling to you and over time, can dissolve whatever dense energy forces are in your body, mind and spirit.

"So Metta is to dilute the dense forces?"

It is not to be narrowly good because even that is another set of karma. That will just introduce a different set of karma that does not cancel out the heavy karma present. To know the spirit you have to bring through pure energy—To identify yourself with Metta.

"How does one cleanse oneself?"

First, you associate yourself with purity. If your karma is not diluted of greed, there is absolutely no prospect of enlightenment or purification and therefore the whole process of cultivation is a waste.

"This is such a difficult idea for people to grasp. Metta doesn't have a body or form—It is not a person but is something akin to spirit that has no embodiment. How can Metta be anything more than a feeling?"

It is a form of vibration. We know it is there vivid and real. It is not an illusion. The beginner, living in physical reality, has not learned how to recognize this energy. Even though it is so real, to the uninitiated or the ignorant it's like showing an illiterate a book to read. But for those who have been schooled and comprehend the language it becomes second nature to read it.

But consider a person who complains that life is sorrowful, full of troubles, illnesses, family, job, financial difficulties, etc. Once that person feels the pain, it's high time to learn how to deal with such karma. Just like a person unable to read, if that person feels unhappy about this and wants to do something about it, then begin to learn how!

What we are saying is this—Everything eventually functions as energies. Spirit is an energy manifestation. So is karma an energy that manifests to cause problems. Gradually, energy can be felt and seen. Until then, you don't know what that is all about.

"It seems that you are asking the average person to trade a known personal identity with something that is a non-identity. This is confusing!"

Identity is associated with an ego, the I, or the self, or me. But if you feel you have enough of your problems and you want to fixed them, then it's high time to try a new approach. With the 'I', problems will always continue to follow. With clinging to the 'I', this body is meant to decay. It's the rule of impermanence that counts. How can you know of something better, such as living in a state of non-identity, unless you check this out?

That is the starting point. You have to make a choice. There is a price you pay for every choice you make. With attachment to identity, regardless of its strength, it will break down even in its prime. The opposite side of success can be failure looming. Downfall! Aging is inevitable. Disease is inevitable. Death is inevitable. So if one wants to cling on this precious bodily aspect of oneself that is the price you pay. Those who are riding high on the tide, won't come down to listen. For them, problems are too far away.

But there are those who realize they have had enough of problems and want to start to deal with them. Then we say we have a promising way out that others have found of value.

"To begin speaking about energy, I first talk about transpersonal psychology. Psychologists mostly study personality and the self-identity and behavior. In additional, there is the notion of an inner existential self with a core of humanistic values. You do the best you can, you identify with goodness and help others as you go along. But that's about all—you live your life according to these values and you die."

"Then I continue and say, 'Supposing you isolate yourself in a room and cut your mind from perceptions of the five senses, and all external stimulation. You also try to slow down your mind from thinking. Then you may, for a while, forget about your personality and your beliefs and values. But what is left is not a vacuum. There's something there that you get closer to as you begin the process of shifting into a transcendent state. You can learn more about this inner core— the real you. This experience leads you to know that this is not empty or a vacuum."

"That's how I start. So I propose—let us find out what this energy is. Once shed, our personality and conditioned learning of who we are falls off and we glimpse another kind of consciousness."

The Fiction of Personality

Let me comment on this notion. All behavioral patterns have both good existing with the bad within a person. These are identities that are acquired through the process of learning or socialization. There is of course a basic survival instinct to take care of oneself even at the expense of others. Some could stoop to do things that are harmful to others, and figure out how to trick others to take advantage of them.

People are also exposed to socialization processes, to be good, to take care and love others. But as one goes on, personal needs become stronger and stronger and the evil side may become prominent. In a materialistic society, the bad nature may surface and the survival instinct arises to gratify and enjoy possessions. Inside, there are still urges to conform to social values that are socially approved. But they are mostly suppressed.

But somewhere in the individual, there is a consciousness of a fight. However, normally the selfish side wins. All these, whether good or evil or bad are identities and characteristics developed from experience and learned. Such identities, even those positive values are not good enough from the CFQ perspective. It's still connected to the self or identity concept.

The greatest purity has no identity at all. It's just as it is. The bad and even the good needs to be further purified, and to be dissolved. By sending out the Metta they are cleared out. We learn to take things as it is. This is the pure energy state of expanded consciousness that has no boundaries. Everything is Emptiness. But this emptiness is comprised of things that are not empty.

On the second notion you mentioned regarding isolation from the six senses and complete sensory deprivation, it's impossible to keep a person totally still. In a quiet place, the karma becomes most active. There is even more mental reflection. The karma will function on its own. While theoretically possible, in reality, people cannot be quiet. The karma plays the fool on them. They have a lot of stray thoughts.

They become more antagonized. The person is truly an advanced cultivator, who, when alone, can be at peace with quietness and remain in Stillness.

Part 3:

After a Denver Conference

4

On Experiencing CFQ Energy Healing

On my third visit with Master Yap, I said, "In my first CFQ presentation in Colorado, you showed me how to radiate energy to participants. I suggested to the audience that they feel this energy—feel the relaxation energy. Further on, I expressed the hope that some will feel the benefits of this relaxation energy—their aches and pains may go away and they will feel better. What else is feasible?"

You can also do some demonstrations of healing plus explain the energy principles of letting go. The CFQ letting go process can be performed by the audience. Some may have immediate results. Yes, this is possible provided that we zero in on the principles of letting go. But first you must remove all reluctance/hindrances to let go. People basically feel unsafe if they are not in control.

"What is the problem here?"

Practitioners have to find a way of not holding on to beliefs and concepts that can block the willingness of letting go and experiencing energy. Once they can allow themselves not to hold on to their normal analytical pattern of thinking, then we can do quite a great deal.

Spontaneous Moving

"I'm sure I can come up with the psychological techniques to open them up and to get them to, say, move to let go, including the Qigong exercises you've shown me."

You can convert it into the normal behavioral pattern. A stressful person normally cannot keep still. When that person sits down, he or she will shift about restlessly, shaking legs or yawning. What does it mean? Sitting down, the person is a little bit quiet. Already the karma starts to be naughty, so there is a need to move about. Movement is a very natural aspect of any attempt to be relaxed.

"Yes, when people are standing too long on their feet they start to sway and lean on one or the other leg or stretch out their entire leg and feet."

Yes, but as they go on they have to relax further and further. To get into the deeper tensions they have to go beyond the earlier movements. We then need to go deep into their psyche to let it move out. True, those earlier movements have some intention involved to move. But as you go on to remove the ego, you don't have to bother how you move.

Movements for beginners are necessary. For them, not moving means their tension energy pattern is of a very dense or very hard nature. While they are not moving constantly, when they do stop that means they've hit upon a layer of non-moving tension or are shifting from one layer to another. Yes, participants must feel at ease and be kind to themselves so that will carry on to being kind to others.

"I can reverse the acquisition process of tension accumulation by first helping them to move in a natural way. Then it becomes a natural process for them to let go."

The impact of the workshop can be great once they are willing to move along with us. We say that everyone can benefit from the pure Qi cleansing energy. Of course, the hindrance everywhere is our ego itself. The path is more like an instrument, from which all the past experiences—the multiple identities or egos will speak through. If participants are willing to let go of their ego that would mean they won't just rely on their past learning experiences, or their karma, or their present knowledge. Then the energy can easily move in.

"On the negative side, I agree that the ego is a hindrance—but that's about all each one of us have. This psychophysical impression of self is the sum total of all our earthly experiences and maybe before that. That makes each person whatever and whoever he is. We look at the ego and the karma of each human being as it tries to struggle free to cleanse itself and that is fascinating and meaningful."

The starting point is a willingness to shed the ego or a willingness to let go. Letting go itself should not be intended. It's like, 'So It Is....'

We say relaxation is letting go. But if you use consciousness to think of letting go then it's no longer so in the purer sense.

"Right, I have learned that to be in a creative state, I have to let go of that intention. Once conscious of pushing myself then it's time to let go."

"How would you introduce the notion of qi to the participants?"

In conventional Qigong the idea of qi sensation to experience energy is to begin with various qi activities. One activity is to stand with feet a foot apart holding hands from a few inches to a foot. Pause and then loosen fingers, relax the body and mentally expand their body outwards. As you continue to loosen and relax more and more, you will feel your hands tingling or vibrating, as if pulsating in a magnetic field. Then the space in between the hands feels more solid and turning your hands in unison the space becomes filled with something tangible. Pull it, press it, and actually feel something that is beyond the physical body as an energy field. That itself is an initial evidence of energy itself.

Try this yourself. You can be seated, and be as relaxed as possible. Once you start feeling pulsations, electrical and magnetic sensations, play with this medium by stretching your hands, or pulling at it diagonally. This will give an impression or idea of what energy is about. It is quite tangible—you can actually feel it. That takes 15-30 minutes for most people to sense. The point is to experience feeling sensations beyond the body and appreciate that one's energy is not confined to within the physical boundaries.

But after that we change tack! Most energy healing systems will say at this point, 'this is valuable qi, so keep it.' But we are saying No! This is actually a dilution of your tension. Your tension is now being more diluted, so it has manifested as electrical or electromagnetic sensations beyond the body. What is experienced is tension being melted away. Certainly, it is not pure qi. What is so tangible is not the pure qi anymore.

So for a half hour do the above to instill a sense of what energy is. But eventually make sure you tell them that this is not regarded as good vital energy. But in conventional standards of Qigong practice one tries to strengthen it, try to keep it. For us, we know that this is just another kind of tension. We know this is the melting of tension.

You've created the initial condition to trigger the melting stage of this tension. And eventually, this must be purified. It's not true that the thicker, the heavier, the denser the energy is, the better. It's simply that whatever it is, it is the manifestation of the melting of tension. So it must be released. It's not something you want to keep—Let go!

As you go on there are all kinds of things—the coarser qi sensations, the heat, the cold, the magnetic field, etc. So you can expand a lot on this and other unwinding reactions for the first topic. After that, you can speak about initiation into regular CFQ. Do a bit of introduction on initiation. Then try to give them more about qi. Do something towards a group initiation. Prepare them to sit the proper way. You tune in to initiate them.

You actually have to zero in and talk more about the movement phenomena. Tell them doing movement is not to intentionally create what one wants but rather it's the freeing of the trapped karma, the tension in the body or that thing that cause problems. Put themselves in the state whereby those things become activated and move out and they are better off by what has been removed this way. So therefore don't hesitate to let go of control—let it move and if you are moving let it continue to do so. But at the same time be careful you're not creating intentionally.

"In a workshop format what physical problems can be performed to demonstrate energy healing?"

It is of course easier to select a more sensitive person to volunteer. You loosen them and they will move. That suggestion itself can work. Perhaps you can attach instrumentation to demonstrate physiological changes as well.

"In terms of relaxation?"

Oh, yes. The volunteer's blood pressure can be monitored and you work on the person lying down. Tell them to relax. Not everyone will be moving. But you should be able to show remarkable changes from the instrumentation.

Another easier way is to demonstrate on the whole group. You ask them to be relaxed, to be loose. You are helping them to relax and you're sending them energy. Some of them will be moving. Just be relaxed. Even though they are not moving, it's O.K. Let them be loose and you send your energy over. I'm sure some in the class will move.

Tell them that they will experience different kinds of sensations such as warmth, or heat in the problem area; that the problem may become more pronounced; and they must loosen, loosen to melt the tension away. I will say from 50-80 per cent will be able to experience something. That will be good enough.

"In addition, what kinds of specific problems can safely be treated and responsive so that volunteers can feel immediate benefits?"

For headaches, there can an be immediate change.

"Migraines too?"

Yes. It can be very immediate. Other kinds of pain can be very deep seated. So may not be easy to treat with immediate results.

"What about wrist pains?"

That may not be very simple. It does not depend only on the symptom that manifests here. The symptom can mean a more serious problem or they can be quite minor. If you select headache pains that will be better. You can tell people frankly that this sort of problem can be dealt with in a workshop in terms of rapid healing effect.

"What about chronic fatigue?"

Not in all cases. Some of them are very insensitive to rapid change. The person will only feel the effect after they go home. They might not acknowledge or agree that they are better within the workshop situation.

"What about back or shoulder pains?"

Same thing. Some of them can be very deep-seated. There will be a substantial reduction of pain. They can even feel the pain moving around during the treatment. But they could also be reluctant to admit that it is better.

"What about the manifestation of self-healing?"

The automatic chant of the Mantra itself is self-healing by nature because that will purify the energy and dissolve the tension. But in the tension flushing out process you'll find that all kinds of movements can be manifested. That includes those who are interested in self-healing. You find that since you've remove away the controlling factor of the ego, it can actually manifest as a form of healing ability. For example, self-massaging, acupressure, and all that. Now just allow it to occur. This will take place, and this can be helpful. But don't think that's all there is to healing. What's more important is just to chant the words.

The alternative approach is that instead of doing it on individuals— you do it through the group. You can devise some system whereby you can actually help them to relax silently. At the same time that you are speaking you sent off the healing energy. Help disperse the dense atmosphere. Like what you've done before in your previous workshops—several times and quite well. After that you can actually ask around for those who feel positive results. Ask those who want to talk about it to raise their hands—just explore the sensations experienced.

"I can start off with different types of relaxation and while they learn the relaxation, I can still send my own energy out. So I can build it up from one day to the next."

The important thing is to create a sentiment about the positive effects. That can be easily done if you can target it in such a way that they talk about it before the healing is instituted. Get them excited about it after. Then they become very interested. That's something I don't bother myself with. But a lot can be done about it. Get them to prepare for the positive effect—let them be excited about it before you start.

"So we raise their expectations?"

That's perhaps a necessary strategy to start things off. They feel they will have concrete results. They paid and now they are receiving value for it. Pay they must—otherwise it won't be appreciated and the best result is no result.

"Please describe the various kinds of unwinding experiences during CFQ meditation and their meaning."

CFQ adopts the middle path approach. Explaining too much of the expected phenomena that will happen or expressing them in words is conceptualization. This kind of knowledge hinders the process of instinctive knowledge (knowing from within). It's better to leave it completely for the participant to discover totally on their own. They'll probably discover little initially as they go in and feel drowsy and straightaway fall asleep. After a while, as they go in, they will experience the sticky energy. It's active, it's mobile, and that's precisely how we dissolved negative energy.

The energy is so sticky and so condensed in us that we have to create, by way of our practice, a great number of physical movements. Then the dense forces can be diluted and dissolved. These experiences can be tremendous and vast for a person who practices regularly or continuously each day. No two days of practice are the same. Over different days, there can be a combination of similarities.

Certain days the experiences appear to be the same. If the person is sensitive enough, probably he or she will know the depth of each negative force being released out. Day 1 will be shallower than Day 2 yet appear the same. Also, a number of forces can be worked on simultaneously within a thick mesh of forces. For example, dominant forces on the left are readily sensed and are very obvious to the practitioner. At the same time, lots of things are also happening on the right side that can be observed, such as on the lower body, on the upper body, and elsewhere external to the body stretching to a distance far apart. How much one becomes aware varies from one day of practice to the next.

They are all happening simultaneously and can easily be overlooked. Of course, you can try to organize and structure these different experiences and figure out their implications. But, in every practice session, there is a tremendous number of combinations of energy events occurring.

For now, we can provide some structure as a useful tool for those considering starting to practice. But once a person has started, convince him or her not to rely on memory or told to expect. Tell practitioners to go in and be prepared to accept things as they are on the basis of awareness itself. Detach from whatever is happening. Whatever happens, just observe what goes on like a witness. Detach your Heart. Expect all possibilities and that will help to erase their doubts about CFQ's potentialities.

With doubts erased, they will take whatever things that happen as it is without trying consciously to explain it away. This is actually a very common mistake for students. Something occurs in their practice and they always have their own explanation according to their beliefs. Their most common explanation is,'Just my imagination,' no matter how physically real it is. There is a denial of perceiving anything and non-admission will obstruct further understanding. This repression also obstructs seeing the full scope of what has changed.

Unwinding the Tension Energies

"I told you about my skin problem on the back of my neck. As you worked on it, I went through the unwinding process. You occasionally pointed out what was happening—the kinds of unwinding I displayed and what energy was manifesting."

This was also a consequence of directly intervening to move out the energy. Do you feel the stickiness of this energy? This energy was pulling you down until you appeared to be stuck to the ground. The physical movements released the tension faster.

"You are explaining what I went through to help my understanding of different kinds of tension forces and that has increased my awareness of them. In my own self-practice, what can I expect as I go along further on my own to work on self-healing?"

Yes, you are here with me for only a short time. It's a waste not to tell you what's happening. I will point them out as they occur. But this is not a suggestion for you to imagine that these experiences are occurring. They are real and totally physical. In general, the practitioner might not see what I am describing until a much later time. But by pointing them out they will realize that is what's happening. Otherwise, they may not have the sensitivity to perceive what's happening.

For instance, if you see the glue itself it may be all around the body. You can be within the glue itself or it is three feet from one's physical body. Again, the practitioner might think, 'That's just my imagination,' and denial of this experience is common. It's easy to explain it away—'O my body is very heavy because I haven't had enough sleep.' Pointing things out will help to be more specific to explore the possibility and once pointed out, when it recurs in future practice, will be perceived.

"Expand briefly on what this phenomena is all about."

First, CFQ is a holistic treatment. It goes in throughout the body and attempts to change the whole body at all levels, physically or physiologically. With proper practice, every practitioner changes in

posture and body structure. This tension energy or glue-like phenomena, as it melts out, can be felt physically and, in some cases, it's
so great that it can be sliced off. When that happens the glue moves
away. At other times, the student feels so helpless in the glue. It's
stuck and whatever he does it doesn't go away.

But that's all right, always come back to the detachment of the
Heart and to spreading of the awareness. Make sure that the person
is not trapped within the energy sensation of the glue. One must
stretch oneself evenly into infinity. In other words, what the person
can feel and what is seen are important. But don't be biased against
what can't yet be experienced in the spaces between.

"How does one expand this way?"

It's understood as such. Take things as it is and make sure not to
imagine things. Even though the physical body boundary is there,
acknowledge the truth that it goes beyond. Such boundary is genuine
but you need not have a boundary. You must do away with this preconceived idea of physical reality.

"Why is that?"

Otherwise that becomes a hindrance. Otherwise one is stuck with
the belief that one is just the body and limbs and that anything
beyond that, even experienced, no matter how real, is untrue. That it
is just one's imagination. In their meditation they might experience
their body changing into a bizarre chunk of force energy. But no matter how real that experience, students would deny it, that it is just
their imagination.

This is associated with one's preconceived belief that one's body is
something else. It simply can't be deformed or be a ball of force one
mile in diameter. So they can't accept that what they experienced is
real nor attribute them to something meaningful like the possibility of
a broader concept of oneself. Yes, one's normal concept or belief can
affect one's progress.

"Why would expanding this concept be helpful?"

Because, otherwise it may hold back one's progress by being insensitive to energy phenomena, by being insensitive to the melting-out
effect. That holding back is itself tension. The student won't be dis-
solving tension in the best possible way.

"You're implying that by expanding one's concept of self, one faces another reality where energy itself is the most real part of you?"

When you hold the possibility of opening to this energy component, not only will one progress but also essentially bring in many other viewpoints. Essentially, Qigong practice means the person must be willing to accept the change that now he is dealing with energy. This point is hard to convince.

"Earlier, I asked a question regarding practicing on one's own. Can you elaborate further?"

The risk of practicing alone is just a sense of loneliness. Believe the benefits of the practice. In your case, you haven't been knocked out by this loneliness and you are fully convinced that this practice is good for you. On the question of speed of progress—Yes, it makes a difference practicing here in my Center within a group. It's the closeness of the teacher and the CFQ practitioners. There is a continuous connection. But not being able to come here should not be an obstruction. In your case, you were away from here for two years. Obviously, in this session you were able to catch up with a lot of things that happened to the rest of my students.

Essentially when you practice on your own, certain things happened that you were not quite aware of. Still you continue to progress without such knowledge or awareness. When you come here, the conditions are right and you know you have felt most of the necessary changes in the past three days. So your absence here did not make much difference since you have been practicing on your own. You will catch up. You do progress even though you have been away from here.

Energy As The Essence Of Being

In the normal waking state, a person deals with physical reality. But when one moves into Qigong practice there must be a willingness to accept the notion that one is now dealing with things energetically. Consider breaking off the disbelief of this possibility—that things not in the normal physical sense can happen. One must be willing to explore, to be adventurous enough to explore, and not try to shut it off.

"So if one does that what can you learn about energy?"

The whole idea of the practice is to detach yourself from the problem or from the past forces that have been created (karma) that have attached to the physical body within and without. Free them out of the body and purify them. Now we are saying that whatever physical events that happens have their own energy basis. That means it has been attracted to cause what is happening in one's life.

Whatever is within a person energetically, it is comprised of his or her past experiences but colored by one's perception of these events. It's not a direct one-to-one correspondence between what the person experiences and what actually occurred in meditation. What manifests is that event plus one's imagination of the product. It will be difficult to differentiate between the imagined product and the actual event itself occurring in the past. They are bound together. Energy can't distinguish the difference—imagination is as real as the physical occurrence of that event.

So in practicing one is breaking off the tension energy. We are purifying ourselves by bringing through the good energy. This is the more positive kind of energy so that we can dilute and dissolve away the negative energy. And in so doing, we change the whole course of our life and our health.

"This is a rather unique description of energy. Most people think of energy in terms of physical energy such as electrical, heat, or food."

We are talking about energy that is the life force itself which is much more subtle. Or to be more specific, about the bundles of impurities on the life force or the spirit itself.

"People think of life force as coming from the biological cellular processes of the body. You're saying it comes from the spirit—that's a rather different perspective."

Yes, a body without a life-force is a dead body. Science can cultivate cells in a culture and ensure that body cells can continue to live on. But science cannot create a living person.

"But some already claim that they have—like a test-tube baby or cloning an entire animal."

That itself is not the same as creation. It's just that science can make use of the basic elements of life and put them in different conditions to create its growth.

"Yes, scientists do not claim to be God."

The conditions for carrying on life is already there. That can continue on its own. So spirit doesn't end there. Is does not end even when the person is dead. The law of conservation of energy means that it will go into a certain transition and change its state.

"In CFQ you hold that the Qigong mentor initiates the student by transmitting energy directly to the individual?"

Attempts on energy practice is different from learning to play a sport which are all physically demonstrable. Energy, to the uninitiated, seems unreal—it's not physically there. They have to find out and experience it. That requires direct energy transmission to help them find out and so the mentor relationship is very important.

I put in the energy and it starts to work on the student. This transmission process can be very important. After the first day of initiation of a new student, normally I feel very weak, drained much more than a regular healing session. In a healing session, no matter how old or weak the patient that's still hard work doing treatment but I don't feel exhausted.

In the initiation session, I am mentally exhausted. My calves ache, my legs feel so weak that I have to kneel down. To teach one new person involves certain element of preparedness to help the novice's karma. In terms of healing, yes, you are helping to dissolve the student's karma or helping to cleanse the impure energy. That is by using Metta to free or cleanse away karma. Then the actual Mantra can be properly and directly transmitted to the newly initiated. Also, in initiation there is an unspoken commitment to help the student to carry his or her karma as it exists and to see to the student's progress that includes future karma.

"So there's a permanent bond?"

It seems that way. I don't fully understand this point but it's much more important than I previously thought. There is a real genuine weakening feeling.

"How shall we end the class?"

Well, make sure that if they're moving strongly that they also detach from it. If it gets too strong make sure they are not preoccupied with their movements. It's not difficult to control. But ask them not to be too excited or frightened by the movements. If they're frightened they'll try to control the movements but they may even become stronger. Cool them down, tone them down to be more relaxed and the movements will be manageable.

But they also go through a period shifting from a lot of movements to then having less movements. Then they may experience violent strong movements followed by mild movements. Make sure they don't conclude abruptly in the middle of strong movements. Let it tone down a bit first. Then the practitioner must intentionally tell oneself to get out of the meditative state. That means to slow down, to stop, and to get yourself out of it. So give them 30 seconds or so to get themselves out. Once stopped, if the body resumes moving, you've got to emphatically tell them to quit. That means in terms of mental activity you come out fully awake—in the awakened state.

The Meaning of Mantra

"CFQ energy healing places great importance on reciting the Mantra you transmit. What is the significance?"

When you use the Mantra you have to explain to them the true meaning of the Mantra. Why is it we don't use words like God or Buddha? Such words have become adulterated by people with different intentions who have varying degrees of understanding coming in to it. And anyway it is not our purpose to overly emphasize religion. We emphasize talking about health care benefits. So we use in our Mantra a few words in Mandarin that commonly signify all that is good.

"The Buddha became enlightened. Did he use a Mantra? Where does Mantra come in for the Buddha?"

People have different inclinations. Some by nature are calmer while others are tenser. People during Buddha's time were definitely more relaxed. Today, they are much more materialistic with more needs, temptations, and stress in life. So by nature it's easier for people in earlier times to click into detachment of the Heart. What matters is detachment of the Heart. Make sure that the Heart does not participate with all of life's events; does not participate in the thoughts; does not participate in the problems. Detach from them as they come.

Bear in mind also that the Buddha, before enlightenment, participated in many types of meditation, until eventually he found that none could solve his problems. At that point of time, naturally it was disheartening and because of this disheartenment, he literally adopted a let-go attitude. So determined did he become that he let go of all physical methods of emancipation.

"So at some point, even the mantra is not needed and you let that go?"

It's necessary until some particular point.

"Did the Buddha used mantras to teach?"

The Tibetan tradition always use mantras. And in pre-Buddha times, there were people who used mantras. I don't know precisely whether Buddha teach mantras but mantras are mentioned in many Buddhist texts.

"But those are much later influences, say from China?"

Mantra is more Tibetan. But is also used in Theravada in South-East Asia. Perhaps in the past there was no need for mantras as the problem of detachment of the Heart did not arise. People living in an era of simplicity of life and simplicity of mind tended to be more committed in what they do when meditating—they put all their Heart in when they meditate.

Today's circumstances are different. You ask people to sit down to do meditation but in their minds they are thinking ten types of things that they want to do at the same time. They are even ambitious in their expectations of what meditation can give to them. 'I meditate, I put in x number of hours, I must achieve x number of rewards.' They are more calculative in their intention.

We know that what causes problems is actually within the mind itself causing physical deterioration in health, disease, and aging. One needs to be detached from the burden of our stressful past experiences—that's what you are. That will only bring betterment—You become relaxed. But you can't claim to be more relaxed when you don't detach from your usual mindset, at least for a certain period of time. Set out a certain time for meditation—just try to detach yourself from what is in the mind, from what is in the physical.

"Right, but isn't what one does with the mind outside of meditation just as important? I am trying to let go of some problem but it proves to be difficult. But by shifting to the Mantra, I find its easier to let go of some depressive thoughts."

Yes, this is concrete evidence that the Mantra helps you to detach from the problem and helps you to be more relaxed. If you're not detached you can never be relaxed. It's like, O.K.—I have a thought but who is thinking? No, precisely you are not thinking. It's the thought that is thinking. It won't work to just say, 'Stop, stop, stop!' The more you want it to stop, the stronger it gets. But when I do something else, that does not give the thought the opportunity for those problems to linger on.

Also, a person during energy meditation can become entangled in the movements as these movements become stronger and stronger. That means the Heart is moved and becomes involved in the movements. At that point, the person cannot remember the Mantra. You have to speak the Mantra softly. Remind the practitioner to detach— to give his or her innermost intention back to the Mantra. Tell them to take it out on the movements. Tell them that they are not the movements. The movements are irrelevant and just move but don't become absorbed by it.

"But still the thoughts and the karma is so powerful, I feel powerless to stop them. Even the Mantra is but one tool to balance all those powerful thoughts. So it's easy for me to lose the battle."

Ah, it depends on your level of cultivation, ha ha. Yes, what we are working against is the near infinite problems accumulated through our life since birth. Our past experiences shape one's character—way of thinking, kinds of behavior, and ambitions we desire to achieve. These are literally very powerful.

If you're ambitious, you're certainly not greedy. It's just that the resulting tension has been built up. So it just goes on and just knocks you out at the least suspecting time. Trying to stop unwholesome thoughts and behaviors, or telling yourself not to do it, you end up not sleeping through the night. Now to face the ambition, there is the Mantra for you, to detach from that thought. In the process, you're actually diluting that obsessive ambition, that depressive thought itself.

If you have a high level of cultivation, it's powerful enough. You tune into the Mantra and you can literally see the force and you can actually melt it away. You see the force which can be a big chunk or a big cloud. Within the cloud are the messages you are thinking about, that have been disturbing you all the time. You see the cloud melting away—it's almost like infinity.

Although you are powerful, the cloud is also tremendous. You see big chunks literally cleared off. But in the next split second beyond that there are still plenty more. In one large chunk, there are hundreds of thousands of forces that come together. These are recurring forces that you literally have to break off one after the other. The advanced cultivator, in one hour, can break off a hundred or even a thousand of these tiny folds or lines of force. But there are still plenty beyond that. In the end, they become manageable and literally become fewer.

"But I haven't actually seen such forces or folds. Does that mean I have not developed even an iota then?"

Seeing itself is one of the aspects of practice. To begin with, the conception of seeing this as something special itself prevents one from seeing properly. For example, you're relaxed, you are loose and as you close your eyes, it's not totally pitch dark, right? It's also not as light as when you open your eyes. There are some shades, a tinge of color pattern that is often there. Just go ahead and discover what they are. As you become more advanced, you'll see chunks of it and you'd see the messages in it.

"For me, characteristically, within seconds of closing my eyes my mind is thinking of something. I am not looking, very quickly after reciting the Mantra I have one thought or another."

For you, perhaps you should shift attention from the thought or idea. Instead of seeing the forces in the force field, try to see the stray thoughts. See yourself in the stray thoughts. Try to see yourself in the Mantra and remind yourself you are meditating. You are doing the Mantra but at the same time as stray thoughts are happening, try to know what they are. You are detached, you are not within the stray thoughts. That means don't follow the thoughts but let the thoughts go.

Let the thoughts happen since the innermost intentions, the Heart itself is with the Mantra. Now your Heart is unmoved. It's in the

Mantra. You are an observer of all the stray thoughts. You can literally see your stray thoughts.

"I see, I see."

Imagine you can literally see the stray thoughts. In the past, when you were thinking you were within the thoughts. So you didn't see anything. Now you will discover that you are probably disturbed by the stray thoughts. You will try to pull yourself out but you won't be able to. Why not? Because you have not detached your Heart properly into the Mantra. Once you detach, you know you are doing the Mantra. Then you can actually see whatever thoughts you have.

"The problem is I like the thoughts. They are interesting creative thoughts related to questions I have. But once I remember, I shift back to the Mantra. But the thoughts come back in some other form again."

The trouble is you like the thoughts very much, haha!

"Yes, they are very useful and helpful in my work."

So that means your choice at that point of time is in the stray thoughts. Your choice is not in the Mantra although you may be trying to do the Mantra.

"Yes, the Mantra helps to let go of the stray thoughts briefly but they come back in a more creative way. Stray thoughts after a while become stale so I naturally refocus on the Mantra to let go of those used thoughts."

That's why you don't see the forces or the thoughts! At that point of time, when you were meditating where were you? Where were your innermost intentions? It's in the stray thoughts.

"Yes."

It's not in the Mantra. So until you are ready to detach yourself you'll never see the thoughts. In between, if you do come back to the Mantra, when you do decide to be with the Mantra, when you are not the thoughts, then you'll actually see the thoughts.

"I think sometimes I do see the thoughts but then I quickly move back to the Mantra but not for long."

At least you have some experiences in that area. In the seeing there can be messages, words, in pictorial form, in a chunk, in a mess, different lights shifting. It's busy out there—a very undescribable phenomena. You are not fully prepared to detach and come out of it. But still you see something of these forces in between. What's important is to remove your Heart from the stray thoughts. You are no longer those thoughts. Another force is waiting to come by and you give it that opportunity to come in. So that the next time you choose to be in the stray thought, Poof! you're in another thought and you go into another sequence.

"I feel happier when I am extending the Mantra or when I am extending the merits to the surroundings. I mean it seems there are two phases in my meditation. One is when I recite the Mantra for myself. At other times, I feel that I'm reciting the Mantra for the benefit of others. Then I seem to feel better, lighter."

Does it occur to you that sometimes if your meditation form is to recite for yourself that it will be hard for you to extend? At other times, when you find that you want to extend, it might be more effective to recite for yourself. Do you experience that?

"Yes, sometimes it doesn't work."

That depends on the resistance, the karmic resistance of it. If you are bound in, you can only recite for yourself and you find that elsewhere it's blocked. But if you're not being blocked it extends out and that itself is visible. When you spread the merits you can sense and see that.

"Yes, when I focus on doing the Mantra on myself all I can sense is my thoughts."

If we think about it maybe we are not doing the thinking! Things are already happening. We are not actually doing the thinking. You say, 'I am thinking of extending the merits.' But no, once you're freed from your entanglement, at that moment you become more open during the extension outwards. At other times, this is prevented—the tension blocks you from extending. You find that you can recite only for yourself. So instead of saying that you're doing it the condition is that—it happened!

"I assume that although I think I am doing it, it's the thought energy working itself out and I just follow it."

From Tension to Stillness

"You spend a lot of time talking about Stillness. On the surface it looks like a conflict or at least a different emphasis in CFQ in comparison to the moving out process."

Of course, one doesn't always have to move and Stillness is not moving at all. If one is moving, it's very hard to see how one has reached Stillness. To be clear, we divide our essence into two aspects. One is the body itself and the other is beyond the mind which is the spirit. In attempting to go into Stillness, first a person has to deal with karma that is already in full swing. All life experiences in the past is now taking its course in generating future events. In order for this link to be changed, the potent forces which have already accumulated in the body have got to be released. In the process of releasing it, we cannot say, 'Don't flow along with the movement of the physical body itself.' That would mean you would not have effective cleansing.

The deeper and shallower elements are all in one. That means they move around together. Detach from the mental aspect or the deeper aspect of things into Stillness. That is very important. Once you get detached you allow the physical body to move. That causes an effective karmic cleansing process. When all the karma is cleansed eventually there is Stillness of the body and the mind. It's like everything is in harmony. But before that the body has got to move.

"So you're separating Stillness in relation to the spirit whereas karma...."

Yes, we're saying that spirit is more important. But the spirit is nowhere to be found because it's all been covered or bundled by the karma. So you separate out and put the spirit back into Stillness and let the karma move out. Eventually when all the karma is cleared, you will experience the non-movement or Stillness of the body and the mind itself. That's truly the advanced stage of cultivation.

"In other forms of meditation such as Zen, Stillness is cultivated from the beginning. Is forcing the body to be still premature?"

Yes, I agree that's a major setback. The concept of karma may not be properly understood in Vipassana or insight meditation. They rely on theoretical knowledge of karma. They don't suspect that karma can be so physically connected to us. The meditators are supposed to experience things for themselves. But if one does experience Stillness readily that is probably due to personal karma rather than the practice itself. Most people, however, with their karma in full swing, will move along with their karma and in terms of knowledge they will interpret things according to their past experiences. That means that they are flowing along with that existing karma.

"But, I can see others refuting what you are saying that you're adding on something outside Buddhism?"

Buddhist practice does not prevent a person's body from movement. Eventually one will become blissful. Buddhism says that all creations or formations are from the Heart itself. So if the Heart is not properly occupied, one is not able to get any effective karmic cleansing. Because of the Heart element, karma is created. So if you want to cleanse the karma, you've got to start from the Heart. But Heart itself is actually nothing until it stops carrying on and on in all its functions.

However, if you use your ego to interpret meditation, then movements are considered wild and even scary. Precisely then, you forget that the Buddha taught you to do away with the ego to attain the state of non-self.

"How do you relate that karma to releasing through physical movements?"

All karmas are creations from the Heart and once created it bundles itself into the spirit, in the mind, and everywhere in the body. So one is not able to immediately detach the Heart into Stillness. You need, at the same time, to give it some work and that work must be so monotonous that's not supposed to create any excitement at all. That itself is Stillness. It is a form of monotony.

The purpose of the Mantra is to give work to the Heart and this work is to generate good energy that is of karmic cleansing nature. Since the Heart is now being occupied, the work done by the Heart itself is by nature karmic cleansing. This means the Heart will be able to spread the Metta to the karma within the spirit, mind, and within the body. And that itself, because of the melting effect on the karma, causes physical body movements.

"Is this mentioned anywhere in any Buddhist text or ancient sutra?"

We base our practice on the Heart Sutra. But Sutras are not manuals for training with specific instructions. The Heart Sutra talks about Emptiness or voidness. That means, in whatever situation, whatever it is—let that be it.

"This book that you suggest that I write—What is the objective?"

I believe that it's an extremely valuable book, in the sense that it will point out the responsibility of a person. It will suggest that one is responsible for one's problems and begin to do something by changing one's attitude. You can also discuss at length the conducive attitude for healthy living. That itself is of tremendous help to humanity. The book should suggest what needs to change.

"Don't most health books try to do this anyway—remind readers of their own responsibility to take care of themselves?"

This book will be different from others in the sense that you will bring out a true story and explain the psychology of it within the true story. Other books only conceptualize it—if you behave or do this you will be healthier. Yours should appeal to the whole person rather than the intellect. Maybe then there's a greater possibility of learning and a change of attitude that can make this a better world. Even a reduction of the tendency to blame others for one's problems is great.

Part 4:

After a Bangkok Conference

5

On the Ultimate Cure

"I have completed some workshops integrating health psychology, meditation and energy healing in Thailand. In previous trips to your Qigong Therapy center I have seen how you treat patients and their amazing cures and recovery. Many of them suffer from chronic illnesses and some appear to be far too gone to have much hope of recovery. Can you identify some recent cases and how they fare?"

There's this young man, age 32, who came to me two months back. Since age ten, he has Type I diabetes and has taken insulin shots for the past two decades. He was in very poor health condition. A year and half ago, he had gangrene of the legs and one big toe dropped off. Both legs were totally blackened, in pretty bad shape, and in danger of being amputated. But he decided to defer surgery and instead he went to the hospital for daily dressing. Fortunately, the diabetes was in control but he had to bear with the pain and the discharge for the past 18 months.

His parents, aunts, and many relatives are all my patients. It's a big family but this person wasn't at all a believer in my treatment. He had stopped work since the gangrene problem and finally he had no other choice but to try me out—in desperation. Ha! My standard kind of patient. When he came to me his face was swollen. The first 4-5 sessions produced impressive results. After the first session, he went home and reported he had such good appetite and sound sleep. He slept for most of the entire day and night. After the second session, the swelling on the legs subsided and the blackened areas on the thighs, all the way down to the feet, were showing cracks. The skin became lighter. After 5-6 sessions, the open wound on the gangrenous leg dried up and began to heal. I doubled up and gave him twice-weekly sessions because of the seriousness of his condition. But he was in a dark mood, felt resentful, and his poor appetite returned. His sleep was fitful and he seemed to have reverted back to the condition before treatment. It stayed this way for two weeks.

Then something strange happened. One day, he got up in his home and seemed to have lost all his memory. He complained that he couldn't recognize anyone. The family panicked and despatched him to hospital. His doctor told the family that the amnesia resulted from brain damage due to his diabetes, that his problem was not treatable, and would deteriorate quickly.

That day they couldn't get hold of me but by the next morning I went to the hospital to see him. He was staring blankly and even when I started to work on him he didn't recognize me, his parents, or anyone around him. He didn't even have a clue where he was—everything appeared to be an absolute blank. I worked on him for half-hour and went home. The moment I reached my Center, his wife called to say that he was out of it—his memory had returned completely! He was discharged from the hospital the second day and looked and felt better than ever before.

"How do you explain this phenomena?"

When these powerful disease forces or heavy energy leave, it literally knocks out consciousness. If not dealt with properly, a person may not get back his memory. My patient's doctor was puzzled over how he had recovered and questioned him during several routine visits. He did not tell his physician how he was treated by me as he was afraid of being laughed at. This is typical of some of my patients who feel ashamed of coming to me and be known by others as seeking 'weird' treatment.

"Tell me again—this is a kind of reaction to the energy that you sent in?"

When his tension was released, too much was stirred up. Well, in his case, you couldn't release it bit by bit. The forces are so strong and at quite a dangerous state when I started treatment. The poisons were everywhere. Note that he has never really accepted my treatment. He was forced by his aunt to receive my treatment because she paid his expensive hospital bills and she decided that mine was better and a whole lot cheaper. But my new patient obliged with ridicule. While receiving treatment from me, he kept praising all kinds of other treatments including herbs, shamans and mediums, crystals, etc.—a long list indeed. And despite having tried many of them without any success, he insisted that these treatments worked for his friends. I became discouraged to the point of wanting to terminate treatment if not for his aunt who pleaded to me to continue.

During CFQ treatment, his body was shaking and jerking physically because of the release of tension forces. But he held on very tightly to disallow this from continuing to happen. He even bragged about how he was able to do so. But when he went home, the movements would erupt when he least suspected it—as he was resting idly, reading the newspaper, or sleeping. As he started to shake vigorously, he panicked as he could not control them. He admitted these occurrences to me and I advised him against holding back but instead to allow himself to release the movements fully. I also said that they would gradually stop when all the necessary tension movements are manifested.

He was still reluctant, and over time he seemed to have devised a way of preventing these movements from occurring—he thought that was an interesting game to play despite my repeated warnings. When he felt much better, I encouraged him to go out for some exercise, to take an easy stroll daily, as walking can improve blood circulation and to give him an activity to occupy his idle time. Besides that, I asked him to help out in his parents' food-stall business and in house-keeping. Instead, he said that he enjoyed sleeping and what I suggested to him was boring and tiring. I replied that he was not really resting lying in bed the whole day but day-dreaming. He was dwelling on his symptoms and aggravating his problem.

These adverse attitudes made treatment extremely difficult and consequently he suffered unnecessarily. You see, my treatment works even on the strongest critics, but when they create conflicts and resist the healing process that cause unnecessary pain. Normally, I will not treat such non-believers who are actively trying to sabotage the energy healing.

A Family of Diabetics

"How does he feel about your treatment now?"

He is still very indifferent despite the fact that his insulin shots are half the usual dosage. You see, his father had 20 years of diabetes too with constant ringing in his ears. The father's problem deteriorated 4-5 years back when he started to have delusions. He hallucinated during the Buddhist Vesak holy day. I cured him of it and took about once a week for a year to do this.

"What about the diabetes?"

The diabetes and hypertension vanished in the process. So now he has stopped all medication since he has no more diabetes or hypertension over the past three years. He is an old man and retired. Now it's the son's turn.

Well my old patient also has a younger son too. Some two years back, he had a motor accident and broke his thigh bone. The surgery required installing a steel plate. However, things went dead wrong after the operation and he did not wake up and instead fell into a coma. Perhaps it was a reaction to the anesthetic. The doctor's prognosis was that he would remain in a coma permanently and at best kept in a vegetative state. They didn't call me right away—only after a month later. I went to the hospital and started working on him. Suddenly we heard him scream that his leg was hurting. He woke up and the first thing he did was to reach for food. Then he demanded to see his girlfriend. All the time he was still on an I.V. drip. He was discharged from the hospital three days later.

"I am surprised that his parents didn't call you earlier."

I am still only the last resort.

"They are lucky that you are here."

The following day I met the young diabetic patient. I quickly saw that his legs had healed and only some scabs remained. He walked with a slight limp but otherwise looked normal.

Healing the Terminally Ill

"Have you worked on other comatose patients successfully?"

As I have illustrated in the family of patients, even in a coma, the person can be revived. The comatose person is aware but can't apprehend the environment. It appears to be very distant. Most of the time, the mind is busy with a lot of dreamlike activity. This situation is not static and the person may drift back into greater awareness or consciousness of what's happening around them.

"People in a coma can be taught how to communicate such as blinking their eyes or squeezing their fingers."

Right, even in a coma, they are busy. They just can't get out of it. They are locked in certain patterns. This is precisely the same for people who are up and walking around! Well here's my opinion of CFQ's healing value. Despite all the enormous benefits demonstrated in CFQ, I feel it still has not reached the full potential which is tremendous. It depends on how far I can let go. I wish to illustrate with a recent patient I worked with, barely two months back, who suffered from a stroke. She is 70 years old and in the stroke she lost consciousness. After five days in coma at hospital the family was asked to take her home for her last moments.

So the following day a coffin was ordered. Some of her relatives have received treatment from me. They convinced the old lady's children to invite me to treat her. So I started working on her on the night of the sixth day. This was her condition then: Her eyes were wide open, blank with the whites like a dead fish, eyes totally rolled up. The tongue was totally dried and stuck out. She was really dying.

After the first session, the next day the tongue rolled back in her mouth and tears came from her eyes. She regained consciousness. She recognize people who came to visit her and she sobbed. When asked to blink to show understanding, she could do that. After 15 sessions in barely two months, she began to move her body in bed. She continued to improve in mobility and was able to move both arms and legs and I felt that prospects of full recovery were excellent.

"You're saying this is no ordinary case and that without your intervention she would not be alive?"

Yes, when I first saw her, she was gasping her last breath. The doctors had given up and said she would not have lasted three days at best. And I only saw her two days after that pronouncement. The family had already prepared for the funeral. I am citing this case to say that CFQ treatment seems to have restored life in the dying woman. It's so powerful that it's scary.

"Something tells me that the woman is not fully recovered."

Uh-huh. At first her rate of recovery was excellent. After about 20 sessions, she could sit on a reclining chair to watch videos—in the past her whole body was totally limp and would slide down. By now, she had some movements in all four limbs, she could make a lot of sounds which were not yet comprehensible. She could sit up in a car to be driven around.

But, don't forget her stroke was extremely severe to the point of total paralysis. So, I suggested that further treatment should continue at my Center rather than my continuing to do house calls. I normally give treatments only in my Center but made an exception in her case because of many repeated requests from her relatives who were former patients. However, the old patient did not turn up for the appointment. I rang up to ask what happened (something I rarely do—chasing after a patient). In her case, I had full confidence that I could help in the total recovery of her physical and mental abilities. Her daughter responded that no one was free to bring her to the Center and went on to say that the mother's condition had not been improving anyway!

Predicting Recovery

"Is treatment success predictable?"

Yes, it is predictable. Even for those extreme cases that have not responded well to conventional or other treatments, we still have been successful. But of course we are talking about so called hopeless or terminal illnesses. The ordinary sicknesses are not much of a challenge. In tough cases, our treatment still works provided the patients give us enough trust to persevere in treatment. Most patients give us less time than they would for normal medical treatment.

Even in alternative physical treatment such as acupuncture using needles, they are willing to give months for it to work.

"I guess I know why. Your Qigong treatment is completely non-physical. You are just standing there waving your hands or sitting quietly. You don't use chemicals, herbs, needles, nothing at all. So how can what you do be really effective?"

Today in doing treatment, I sit down without even waving my hands except at the beginning and in concluding the treatment. I sit behind them and they are lying down. I close my eyes and tune in. That's all.

"So you are in meditation when you do healing?"

That is precisely how things work. I work on the life itself and by freeing the entanglements in the life force, repairs to the physical body takes place on its own, and the patient recovers. All other treatments whether using medication, drugs, surgery, herbs, acupuncture, etc., work externally on the physical body and have, at best, limited effectiveness. Most medical or health professionals see you as a malfunctioning body to be fixed much the same way as a mechanic would repair a car.

However, if the body is the car, the driver is your life or spirit. Yet when something is wrong with your life, you blame the car. So you think the solution is to work on the car. You figure the car is pretty empty and you try to stuff up the interior and end up choking the driver. And so in no time, the life in you says, 'Bye!' and leaves. But there's any number of people who will ridicule the very suggestion that a living being exists as a body with a spiritual side. But I insist, your body has a wonderfully sophisticated built-in self-repair feature that knows exactly what to do provided you free the 'driver' instead of burying and suffocating that energy. The non-physical way that I am laying out is the only maximally effective way. That is, opening from inside out, flushing all the way down.

"Potent enough to rid one's life of all biological and psychosocial trauma?"

That is true holistic de-stressing with one generic cure for all ills. Conventional physical treatment, no matter how superior it claims to be, is added on as an external input. But in reality this is adding new stress that entangles, although one may get quick relief as the symptom becomes hidden. Even relaxants enhance stress and in the long run, the dosage needs to be increased. The net result of the suppression effect of holding on is to add more stress to exacerbate the problem further.It is unrealistic to expect transformation in people. A student may have a good day in CFQ meditation meaning that cultivation has changed his condition. His health has changed for the better, and he is advancing in spiritual development, and all that. But don't expect people to change that fast—they are still locked into their own patterns of thinking and behaving. They are not willing to sacrifice or let go of their precious ways for serious cultivation. Most people wish to live long, stay healthy, and young, but are much less willing to pursue a commitment to cultivate letting go.

"What's the happy median?"

We suggest that we have a method for them but if they don't try it out.... In my own situation I have to balance between doing more to propagate CFQ and letting things unfold. Options for me are limited in the sense I can only practice very hard daily. If someday CFQ takes off, I actually will have to go through multiple tests to verify its efficacy. That's my role. But as far as healing is concerned, nothing is a mystery to me. Wealth or fame is too bothersome for me. That's letting in more tension. I am primarily concerned with the art itself. To be more relaxed.

"Yes, I know you live simply and unpretentiously in a small house with your wife and three small children. You have cut down on the patient load to devote more time for your own meditation. And as for your Center, you have a big mortgage to pay off!"

As said before, each person is locked in their own karma. It is this karma that determines what they will do next. To do something new also is determined by whether their karma allows or accept the change. For example, someone will start off liking CFQ, but their karma comes in and closed them off and they may do something else. On the other hand, karma can mean that people are afraid to fall sick and die. But that itself is a good karma connection that can pull them toward CFQ. But their commitment to continue is another thing. One might feel unmotivated to continue.

Some former patients might dispute this but we don't feel concerned or necessary to defend or challenge others. It's futile to even try. Say a person has a 20-year health problem. He comes in for nine months and receives 40 sessions of treatment and he gets cured of his problem. Yet he doesn't believe that you've helped him. With each healing session, there are strong positive effects—some are even agonizing, others very pleasurable. But once treatment is over, he forgets the benefits.

"Perhaps CFQ by not claiming anything specific will not be given the credit even if the person is cured."

Many claims are made by other Eastern healing systems making many specific promises. But how much of these can be delivered—maybe one person out of a thousand claims gets results? However, that person becomes very excitable and the news spread to a thousand while the disappointed ones says nothing. But CFQ would look at this excitement of the achievement itself as a form of tension which is undesirable.

Some of the local healers here often mention my name in comparing themselves. They say it's not possible that I can do continuous healing for this long a period. They refer to themselves as having better and more powerful energy—and their healing is much more effective. Still they loudly acclaim that with one touch the person is instantly cured! Such a phoney healer gets a lot of followers in the short run.

In the past, there were half a dozen such healers that I know who lasted a couple of years and now have mostly disappeared. Of course, they made a lot of money, a few even became rich. Eventually, such people disappeared because a lot of promises they made could not be delivered. So the Master runs away and the students are left in the dark.

There are ways of convincing others that we absolutely won't—Stir up a lot of grandiose expectations about one's system, or put up an impressive Center with appealing or aesthetic surroundings. These quacks get publicity by constantly talking about the wonders of their system. They put up sensational demonstrations and performances in the public eye even if it has nothing to do with Qigong. For example, martial techniques of astonishing power. These performances are convincing—people get excited, and they go away talking about how powerful they and their masters are, even though they've only learned Qigong for a few weeks. But that itself is a form of tension creation as they literally worship what they are doing. With such devotion they give undue credit to their training. It does have the required effect of stirring vulnerable people to listen to them. But there's no way they can fulfill them. The bottom line for such people is that they get rich.

Now here in my Center, we don't try to create such a devotion since, in the long run, this leads to disappointment. Our students are mild and quiet even though they might start off with a boastful attitude. Basically this is a CFQ effect as well. We work on ourselves and it delivers but we don't have to boast. Boasting may not lead to achievement—too much energy wasted talking and telling others about their imaginary achievements.

"Many methods attract a lot of interest on the short term—like a fad but on the long term fades away."

Right, they create the worship effect and has a tremendous attraction. We absolutely make sure that we don't make outlandish claims but stick to the truth. Some Qigong practices claim to enhance sexual power to attract those who want this. But CFQ has a generalized health impact—and sexual potency can be a by-product. That, however, is not the goal of cultivation. I had one young patient who was totally impotent. After three months of practice he regained this capacity—and powerfully. Another person, after three years of practice, regained youthful hardness. He claims that sex could be prolonged at will.

"Is this because they were much concerned with sex from the beginning of practice?"

No, not necessarily. This normal physiological ability is inbuilt and deteriorates because of tension. If you unwind the tension and become more relaxed, the ability comes back naturally. But when it changes, our students don't make a big thing over regaining their ability.

We are not too interested to be the savior of all humanity. For the time being at least, those with the right karmic connection come to us and we help them to solve their problems. We can't save everyone as we know there are so many limitations. Those who can only be convinced by more sensational masters and claims won't come to us. We won't create the worship effect to draw others in.

"We are the source of all our problems as we are the cause?"

Our well-being depends on how we think, our normal functioning and our behavioral characteristics. Even when there's trauma and negative experiences, the impact depends on how the person takes things. Asking a person to take responsibility is often an obstacle that a person resists. Typically, if one has a problem, someone else is responsible for them. Therefore one can simply rely on medication.

"However, there is some element of truth that everyone is a victim of circumstances. Children are abused or neglected, or exploited."

No, we don't blame anyone for their ills. Asking one to take responsibility does not amount to blaming them for their problems. Absolutely not. Problems start off with what one is born with, continuing childhood experiences, as well as into adulthood. The person may not even realize that what happened is not conducive to health or certain behaviors create harm to themselves. For example, suppressing anger, or that getting angry over minor things will cause so much problems to themselves. If they had been aware, probably things will be slightly different. But by the time you get to tell them about the consequences, they have gotten out of hand or their temper is uncontrollable.

"Yeah, regardless of knowing or not knowing, since the negative emotions are ingrained the consequences will follow."

That's not to say one is guilty, though. When illness strikes, one is just a victim of previous trauma, previous exploitation or one is paying the price for worldly achievements. That person didn't ask for it, but they did take place. So the responsibility now is to remove the causes of present negative effects. One straightforward thing is to take some responsibility, be brave enough to face it, and work on oneself.

In Search of a True Cure

"It seems that full recovery from illness can be obstructed by other non-treatment factors?"

A former patient persuaded a cancer patient to see me. Three months after the complete course of radiotherapy, the cancer had spread throughout both lungs. When he first came for my treatment he had no appetite. After two sessions, the appetite improved. After 5 or 6 sessions, he gave the excuse he had no transport to get to my Center, and stopped the treatment. But still he survived for another seven months.

"How come? He just gave up?'

Um, no. People have their own views of treatment and cure. He certainly was depressed, and he probably felt that the treatment was too slow for him. Even though conventional treatment normally requires regular treatment over years, many people when they come to me grow impatient and feel that the treatment is taking too long. This was the case of my aunt you documented previously. Remember, she was getting results from my treatment but still continued to look for something better. She survived for a year despite stopping treatment and yet when she started treatment with me, she was near death.

You see, you can't change hardcore thoughts. The person becomes the thought itself. We can ask the patient to sit back for the energy healing and throughout our treatment we explain the problem situation and what to expect. Patients in most cases, however, prefer to follow what others have to say about their illnesses or what the majority tells them. It is a rather special person who will listen to an energy explanation of disease causality and treatment modality.

You see, people expect that something physical must be done by the healer to eliminate their disease. The disease itself is the enemy and must be destroyed. If someone comes to me for treatment, I ask the patient to lie on a couch and sleep, while I sit on a chair behind and close my eyes. The person thinks, 'This is nuts! This healer should be zeroing in aggressively to eliminate the problem, not go to sleep himself.' How do I deal with this issue? Make them pay! People measure work done with money and expect value for the money they put out. So if they feel cheated, don't come back. Otherwise, at least, they feel they are receiving a valuable service commensurate with what they have paid!

Then some are really poor that deserve a discount or a free treatment. But it's not easy to figure the truth from what they say. There was this patient with bad arthritic knees who was completely cured after 50 sessions over a one year period. The patient's thigh and calf muscles had fully regenerated, while the shin bones had straightened. Gone was the chest congestion, heavy head, tiredness, pain and insomnia. In fact, in the end, the patient could walk faster than her children and grandchildren. She originally pleaded for a reduced fee and paid a total of less than $400 to me. What a surprise! After her recovery, she came back to inform me that she wanted knee surgery to have new metal joints installed that will give her perfect bionic legs. She confessed that she still had the more than $10,000 she had set aside for the operation prior to seeing me!

Everyone has their own theories and explanations of diseases consistent with what others popularly believe in. The problem is that such a person will be totally shut off from any new ideas or helpful suggestions. Even if the person is willing to listen, the question is how much will seep in? If their illness is rheumatism, the doctors here tell them it has to do with 'wind and water.' I tell them otherwise, that they have to get rid of their tension energies but they don't accept it preferring to cling to the popular belief of wind and water causing the disease.

"In a more general sense, thoughts bring about a particular reality or concrete result. For many, the cause or thought and the result or effect seems to be very slow. For others, the cause and effect seems to be almost instant. They think—I want to be cured—and almost immediately, they are cured. There's no gap between the cause and effect. For other people it never happens, or it takes forever, and they are already dead. There seems to be a time lag between the thought and the manifestation of the result?"

Basically you are referring to the behavioral pattern of the thought itself. Some thoughts are more flexible—that means the person is more flexible. Some people are more rigid—their thoughts are more rigid. You cannot give a new suggestion that they will readily accept as they hold on to their old ideas real tight. They will go all out to defend their old thoughts. Others are open to new possibilities. At least in this case there is scope to tell them what exactly is happening about their illness. But with a rigid person, there's no room to tell him or her otherwise.

"So having the original thought or wish to be cured is not enough?"

Right, unless another series of things are introduced. Say, a person is depressed with some problem. If the individual's thought pattern is open to a new suggestion beyond the notion that he can't be cured then the energy of this new thought, 'I can be cured,' seeps in. This temporarily cuts off the old hopeless thought and the depression is lifted. For the time being, the person's situation is more manageable. The symptoms are considered as less of a problem. But this is not a cure, and we've got to dig in further. So the so-called miracle taking place is really opening up with a new thought so that new energy comes in. This is enough to tip the balance to be healthy. At least to temporarily pacify the negative thoughts or negative energies that create a disease pattern. It helps to calm down the person and not give so much disturbance.

"But there are miraculous cures on record. In France, there's Lourdes—people go there, soak in or drink some blessed water, and become cured."

In some cases, the power of belief can be harnessed. The element of faith can be so strong that something physical actually happens. That faith-power is so strong that such a drastic change happens. Here the energy of faith also co-exists with the original energy of the disease. The disease energy becomes dormant and hidden. If no new factor comes in later on to trigger the dormant disease, it is considered as cured for good. Normally, however, I am quite suspicious of miraculous cures which turn out not to be so.

"I think there is a good reason why there's this buffer between thought and external reality. Without it, all kinds of crazy things could occur. Somebody wants to get rich and that occurs overnight or someone has a destructive thought and there is instant gratification. If there's no gap or buffer that shields the effect then this world will be totally crazy."

Certainly there is a buffer. Thoughts are complex forces—a person is the sum total of all his or her experiences, positive and negative, etc. An individual's mind is not a tabula rasa and the infinite thoughts and past memories become forces within. These serve as a neutralizing effect. They compensate each other. Therefore thoughts don't generally produce an immediate strong effect. But in certain situations, as when a person has such a tremendous belief, these thoughts become more powerful. Basically, people can think of something but at the same time not actually believe in that thought and there's little consequence.

"Just like a passing thought?"

They may try to believe in that thought, but they hit a very shallow limit. Then the intensity dwindles away, and they think of something else which could be totally the opposite. They have doubts, or that it won't work, etc. Take this situation: 'I think I can lift this big sofa up but at the same time there's another thought,'No, you can't really lift that.' One tries to convince oneself, 'I can do it, I can do it,' but the opposing thought is still predominant.

"So, in that sense, does the Mantra works to reduce this buffer?"

Yes, the Mantra is suppose to melt away all the negative thoughts or all the forces that are the source of those thoughts themselves. So therefore it's a purification process. Once one is purified, just turning on the thought is powerful and can have direct effects. There's already no hindrance. There's no more, 'You can or you can't,' and no likes or dislikes. There's no controversy at all.

"So in that sense when you're using the Mantra for healing the effect is instantaneous?"

Yes, just do it.

"You don't have to worry about transmitting or moving the energy from here to there, etc.?"

No, there's no need. Actually, in the process of healing, things are changing—constantly and fast. The energy goes there, and the thought comes,'You have to go there.' Then when the forces move to another place, it also manifest in your thoughts, 'Oh, go to that place.' You think you are thinking but actually the forces are directing you through your thoughts.

"O.K., but there's still some processing going on when using the Mantra?"

Correct.

"But you are not consciously directing or doing it? You are not intentionally creating a certain effect?"

You just carry on without trying to direct your action or thoughts.

To Diagnose or Not

"Isn't diagnosis the first step in all therapeutic interventions?"

When a person sits down for me, I can diagnose the problem from the patient's posture, facial expression, and the physical pattern. I need not have to tune in energetically to diagnose the problem. That's what I used to do. I try to feel, I try to see, and then come out with a certain conclusion or diagnosis.

But I have also found that I can actually be misguided. Because one tends to tune in to the more superficial things while the disease-causing forces exist in endless chunks. What is obvious may not be the most important. Indeed, diagnosis can take the form of tuning in to feel the sensations of a person. If a person has a headache, it's likely that you can also feel a headache. To see and feel the forces, to sense its sensations—these belong to the psychic diagnosis aspect of a healer.

But I believe that this is certainly not good enough and can be misleading as well. So we also have to tie in with the external physical condition of the person. Say the posture of the person, body size, or the complexion—all these denote how one has been carrying oneself around. And that has a greater impact on what one's problem is today. This external appearance does tie in with the psychic diagnosis but not totally. But what we diagnose psychically is inadequate and can only detect the superficial symptoms.

"In Oriental medicine, the pulse is most important to diagnose symptoms before they manifest physically. That of course is important for prevention."

But with CFQ treatment, the changes in the physical signs and the pulse can take place very quickly and drastically. From one session to another, these are totally changed! So we are saying, dependence on pulse diagnosis is still not good enough.

"But what about the notion of diagnosing symptoms before they appear physically?"

Yes, a traditional physician proceeds that way from diagnosis to predict what will likely happen next—but that prediction can never be precise. I believe that compared with checking the pulse we can do more by looking at observable factors and the physical body. For example, a person's posture with raised shoulders tends to have a lot of tension in the upper torso or body. The lifting of the shoulders could lead to hardening on the neck. If you see that the chest is rigid there is high risk of a problem developing. If you look around and find some red spots behind the neck, that person has a high risk of suffering a stroke. This can be quite accurate.

"That's right. I was present when a relative of mine had a stroke. As I comforted him, I found some red spots behind his neck."

"Has the tension built up?"

Yes, it has become hardened. Diagnosis is not meant to be an accurate science. It's only a direction of where the person is heading. I am saying we need not start with diagnosing the new patient. As we do the treatment, we also do the diagnosis to find out what causes the problem. It is also better to listen to the patient directly. Let him tell you his complaints about what he feels. Then we will find out where exactly is the problem.

But anyway that is not our real interest. I mean, we find out because we want to make a comparison with how the patient progresses later on by checking the posture or seeing how the energy system actually changes. We fall back on the principles of CFQ treatment so that we are not too concerned on what we work on first, or what we pluck away later.

We are not concerned—just tune in and work on the person as a whole. We are saying that all problems are just like, well, a pail of rubbish. We don't have to distinguish which part of it causes a headache and remove that or which particular trash causes a stomach ache and take out that part. In fact, we can't, as in effect it's more like a bucket of garbage that's mixed together. So we go in, open the lid, just see whatever garbage there is, and throw all that out. They are all relevant.

But after some treatment sessions, the patient says to us, 'Now I feel better when you do that.' The patient subjectively tells you how things have improved—'My headache is gone!' But we were really not working on the headache.

"You're just removing a chunk of forces?"

Correct.

"So, as you said you let the person lead you in terms of what their subjective symptoms are."

No, not lead but give the patient an opportunity to tell us why he or she comes in. We don't make a judgment. If the patient says he doesn't have a problem—we say, 'O.K., you don't.' It's better this way because eventually we are talking about the person's thoughts or mind that creates the problem. So if someone believes that they don't have a problem, let them continue with that belief. That will be better than trying to convince them otherwise.

We say we are treating all problems as rubbish in a pail or a bin. Everyone inherently has almost every problem or illness. The difference is how the disease manifests, that varies in intensity and degree. But each person has every problem. The whole process of aging itself means that they have every problem.

So it's like saying that for people who have poor circulation, that could lead to diabetes in one or a different problem in another. Which disease depends on other factors, such as what occupation or lack of occupation. So what we try to do is improve the circulation, loosen it out, and just de-stress the person. CFQ is an ultimate method that is non-specific and works for all. We use no set treatment procedure—It just gets to the root of all diseases.

"But it takes years for the practitioner to get to that level of mastery in healing. That's a problem for wanna-be healers. It may take many years, maybe a lifetime, or never."

You can still do it according to your degree of attainment.

"But is it really effective?"

It will still give some degree of effectiveness. You see, nobody knows precisely what a state of cure is. You just have to do it with sincerity—that itself will be a cure. When a person feels better after treatment, that itself is a cure because as you move in you realize that the healing process is an infinity.

Defining a Cure

"What is a cure?"

For us, cure for a 80-year old man could be bringing him back to the state of an 18 year old. Or the physical condition of an 8 year old. I mean, that is not expected of us to pull off. Theoretically, healing here is a reversal process. But how much is a person willing to allow you to do or to work on? How much is the person willing to sacrifice to be cured? How much pain is he or she prepared to endure during treatment to create that effect? Then ultimately we ask—is it morally or spiritually right for the healer to interfere so much?

A person comes to us seeking relief for a problem. So we are doing our job and we do it conscientiously. That's what is expected of us. Full stop, all right? We're not cheating on the patient. Someone comes in and in fact I work on all the person's problems since I look at all the problems as one—they are all like rubbish in a bin. So long as I clean up, the patient has, at the least, a lighter bin. But even the best conventional medical cure today, from the way we see it, is far from a cure.

Say a person has a limp because of sciatica. He goes for an operation and medication. After six months, he or she comes out and says, 'Oh, the doctor tells me the surgery was 100 per cent successful—so I'm totally cured.' But look, the so-called cured person still walks with a limp. Worst still, the whole back and body now becomes rigid. But that's the best medical cure there is! Here in CFQ treatment, even with a very preliminary stage of training, say with 1-2 years of practice, I think such a new healer can give a much better cure than any form of conventional medical treatment.

On your suggestion that our treatment is not specific and that is a weak point, I'm saying, "No, that precisely is our strong point." Remember we are talking about the "method of no-method" and because of 'no-method' it works on all since all problems are interconnected. It is because of this interconnectedness that it cannot be isolated. Isolation itself causes some adverse effect.

Methods are worthwhile in the socially-accepted sense. Methods, however, from the spiritual-philosophical standpoint cannot carry you to the ultimate or optimal state. They are, for us, more like 'flowers in the mirror' or 'moon in the water.' You say you own the flower, but you are actually only looking at the flower in the mirror. Why not look at the flower itself? Perhaps looking at the mirror seems real or more impressive. But as in our finding after examining all methods, they promise more than they deliver.

"I look at this as a practical dilemma. For you healing is everything or a nothing kind of a thing. For someone like me who may aspire to be a healer, there is a need to have some guides. Otherwise, one can essentially only be your student unable to function as a independent healer."

With CFQ practice, there is no such thing as graduation. Other therapies come up with a training approach in stages. But making claims of being at the advanced level is one thing. It's another in terms of how effective. They are probably only promises but nothing valuable in effect.

"Yes, they obtain certificates for their training and are happy."

We don't like the idea of telling a lie. No one can dispute the certainty of birth, aging, disease and death. Yet, we say that human beings aren't that hopeless—much can be done to make our lives happy, healthy, and fulfilling. One can actually jump out from that cycle but to accomplish that requires that you set your target or goal very high. Once you've set the goal, just continue and be committed. Cultivate and 'Just do it' as a way of life. Of course, without sacrifice you don't get anything. That sacrifice is almost infinite.

"This suggest that a healer is not a normal ordinary human any longer?"

The CFQ healer is a healing machine. We don't indulge in personal emotions or cling to likings or who we like to work on. We pay a price for our aspirations. If one is willing to sacrifice to that extent I am sure one can go very far as a healer.

"Yes, that's the price an enlightened healer or bodhisattva, who makes a vow to save others, voluntarily accepts. But what do you mean—no likes or dislikes?"

Be careful not to be too emotionally involved with the patient since that hinders the healing itself. For example, a person coming in who's sick and in a pitiful state. Yes, to sympathize with a person is a natural human tendency. Your sympathetic manner, however, is not sufficient to change their condition. You have to reverse the disease state and change that. For that you need to go through a state that is beyond empathizing.

"Is this because the healer is creating unnecessary tension?"

Yes, you can get entangled in the sympathetic situation. It's easy to get entangled when you tune in since you are tuning into a lot of anger, hatred, etc. You go along being less emotional and that depends on how much you have cultivated your unmoved Heart. That itself will help cleanse off the emotion of anger from the patient. In other words, the emotional state of the patient or the physical state needs to be changed.

"But you have often stated that the most fundamental thing in healing is radiating loving kindness. Isn't that an emotion?"

Compassion itself is not an emotion in the narrow or shallow sense. When compassion comes in, the personal aspect has already been eliminate and is now much broader. Compassion as such has becomes radiant. If there is a personal identity, that energy is no longer radiant. No identity—neither yours or the patient—should be involved.

"But that's difficult to do."

Of course, yes. But the ability to do it affects the result essentially. It is better to be in a neutral kind of situation.

"Right, to make sure that one is always radiant is to let go of one's personal emotions."

CFQ effects on Mind, Body, and Spirit

"You've talked about CFQ in the context of health and aging. But also you have hinted that it can change a person's course of life."

Even one's career, relationship with others, and social problems.

"Tell me how."

Through the practice of CFQ, you melt away the karma or the forces which are the particular negative traps in a person. Once they are dissolved, a person becomes more positive. And being more positive, the individual finds that he or she is opened to a sequence of better future prospects. By being more radiant, the person is open to more fortunate opportunities. By getting rid of certain negative or restricting limited paths one is in, one becomes socially more conscious and understand others needs better.

"So all the gains come from a blanket effect and not a specific effect?"

Yes, this is precisely what is happening to the practitioners and patients in my Center. They find that plenty of changes happen to them. We believe that these positive changes in their lives originate from CFQ.

"You have insisted that physical health and spiritual health are related. You see this very clearly in your work?"

We go in and sense this quite naturally. In our meditation workout, we dissolve and dilute the physical tensions and clear them out. You asked earlier why the CFQ approach is not described in standard texts on meditation. I believe that what is spiritual is also subject to all kinds of speculation and imagination. Many disciplines speak of spiritual development as a belief, trust, or faith in some supernatural being. That itself is a lie. We are saying that spirit is the very essence of life itself.

"Where is this essence of life?"

It's within the innermost intention in us. Because we have this basic intention, we fall into this cycle of life—birth, aging, illness and death. Then there's a continuation as things doesn't stop there. The whole process is an add-on or adulterated process of deterioration. Specifically, in the case of diseases, the tension generated are just added on and on. As people age, they get more and more problems.

Even medical treatment and alternative healing methods use some add-on ingredient such as a drug or herb or when a therapeutic program is provided. In CFQ, through unwinding and the letting go effect, we don't have to promise—the benefits follow the practice. So we are saying if you can effectively stop or reduce the add-on process and go on with the letting go process then you're free of your problem.

Eventually, you see that there is no set of standard criteria for what is good health and what is poor health. It boils down to how one thinks—the quality of one's thoughts in one's mind. If one thinks one is healthy—then one is. We can look at someone and think—he's old and sickly, based on conventional standards. At that stage, it's very difficult to do anything concrete to get him out of his sorry state.

But there's another way—if you can change that individual's attitude. We tell the patient,'Don't indulge in self-pity. There are others who are in worse circumstances.' That could change the person's outlook and mental health. And that brings a lot of health benefits despite one's current physical state. Get the person to accept the situation and still be content and not to indulge in self-pity which could worsen the person's condition to deteriorate very rapidly. Being more open now, the person actually slows down deterioration and that is a pre-requisite for reversal of poor health.

"Just by changing the person's attitude?"

Yes.

"How?"

Well, say the patient has a minor pain—and he stops wanting to move his hands and he feels others must feed him. He stops trying. But once he believes the pain is attributed to his aged condition and thinks: 'I am lucky, most people don't live to 80.' So he's more open that way and thinks, 'Why not? I can still feed myself!' Becoming physically active actually helps him recover or regain complete use of his arms. So there's a scope for improvement in quality of life.

On the outside we might see someone who lives in poverty and we think that's pitiful—the person hardly has enough to eat. But that poor person is contented with his or her lifestyle, thinking, 'I have enough food, my clothes are old but clean. I'm all right.' This person doesn't fall into discontentment and he may be much luckier than many others who are materially better off. The average person has to struggle hard to live. But such people who supposedly is living in poverty don't have to struggle so much to maintain their simpler needs.

"Yes, happiness is relative and often based on comparisons with others. A rich person who compares himself with another with greater wealth feels poor by comparison and grows discontent."

That's the same with health too.

"But if disease is not reversible—how much can be done?"

O.K. Take a patient with a bad heart. We are saying that even with that, physical changes happen that makes him better off. In addition to a conducive attitude, with a certain technique such as CFQ, one can do a lot to reverse a unhealthy state or condition.

"I have read of cancer patients who, having accepted responsibility for their condition, set out to change themselves and thereby regain their health. They face up to the fact that something had indeed been wrong in their attitude, lifestyle, or behaviors. They re-examine themselves and attempt to change a number of things with the result that the cancer also disappeared."

In more severe cancer problems, the time when it manifest is also when the deterioration speeds up to become diagnosed. The person, on being told this, becomes very excited, very restless, generating a lot of worries and finally resigns himself to a no-cure state. He may be having the problem for ten years without knowing it. It could be that he discovers it by chance. The person is in a intense state of fear—like a acute stress response. He thinks he must fix it fast and have to find any available treatment or otherwise the deterioration accelerates to the end.

But as said, the available treatments are always an add-on process. This means that it may be unable to cure a real dangerous disease since adding on worsens the problem—in the long run. The person frantically looks for a cure as time runs out. He may undergo conventional and alternative therapies—which can mess up his system further. The stress alone is unbearable and biologically harmful. This further complicates the situation, even in cases where no cancer is present. The suggestion of having cancer is itself devastating.

"Experiments show that the power of belief—the placebo effect— can actually melt tumors and cure cancer."

Yes, the element of faith shows how remarkable the mind is. So if a person has the belief that he has an incurable terminal disease he is almost certain to die from it. Today, given the negative propaganda about cancer virtually anyone diagnosed with the problem will not make it. The fault lies in the propaganda plus even in the treatment itself. The treatment is not right.

"Earlier, you mentioned the critical role of the spirit not because of religion but because spirit is the basic element of life. So you imply that consciousness itself is more fundamental than physical matter?"

It's saying that physical matter is only one level of reality. True reality so to speak, is spirit that is non-physical. So it must be some kind of consciousness.

"Many people will challenge this assumption."

According to meditative wisdom, that is the truth, that's reality. How does a person come into being? The beginning of life of the physical body comes from nothing that is tangible—a sperm or egg alone doesn't develop into a life form. There must be some life force involved for these cells to develop into a life. For the sperm and egg to merge, the life force itself comes in and then there's physical development. On the other hand, in death the body is still in intact condition but where is the life? The life is nowhere to be found! The doctor will simply say that the heart stopped, the brain died, and so there is no more life. Well, there's more to it than that—a mystery even.

Take our mind and thoughts. Scientists say that our thoughts are stored in the brain. That itself is false—how do these thoughts become organized? It's the ego or self that is involved. Negative symptoms appearing during the treatment are positive signals. But the patient's family may not see this as progress. To start off, they come to me to take a gamble for some quick miraculous cure. But eventually, when they see that a lot of hard work is required, they start to disbelieve and stop coming. They don't see me touching or physically working on the muscles. No surgical measures are performed. No medication is given unlike conventional methods.

"So what is it that works in CFQ?"

By de-stressing to melt away the tension inherent in the body that prevents it from developing normally.

"I hear you and it sounds so simple. But why is it so difficult to accept this, to believe it?"

Well, people like to go for methods and tangible things. My thesis of disease and life is too simple for others to accept. It's just tension and relaxation. People want to believe there's something much more complicated.

"And maybe it goes back to a previous discussion you said that spirit is the innermost aspect of life. But most people would regard this physical body as me."

On the other hand, people also sense there is an unknown. Somewhere in them they also believe in the existence of another kind. It's too vague to talk about and they can't quite comprehend what that is but conflicting views are normal in most persons. It's also scary to talk about something like spirit. If it exists, then it is possible for someone evil to cast a spell and cause a problem. So there's a heavy suspicion of such notions. There is no understanding of the super-natural and so they're afraid of it.

"If something like what you say is true, they're quite frightened by it. It's unknown and kept at arms length. That puts a healer like you at a disadvantage."

That's precisely how the healing works. De-stressing comes from working on the spirit to clear off the burden from the spirit itself.

"Why has nature made it so difficult for humans to find their way out of their predicament in life? Then there's this fear and suspicion of anything that's not concrete."

Humans have special features that other forms don't have. Lower animals live on instinct—they know how to survive and their species' survival depends on meeting their instinct of hunger, seeking out food, procreation, and that's the end of it. Humans also have this basic animal property. But we have these thoughts in our minds as well—that creates, that destroys. Often there are built-in destructive tendencies, for example, anything created in nature is meant to be destroyed. The law of impermanence rules. At the same time because of our free will and free thinking we can do much to understand the nature of existence and try to free ourselves from the whole cycle of life itself.

So that also implies that if we are freed from the body to the non-physical state—then it's easier to understand the spirit. Buddhists say that you have to be born in human form to be enlightened.

"Yes, but is there still non-physical existence or a transition after death?"

There's still the ego that serves as the main control where all the thoughts, the karma are bundled together. We all wish that all the forces, the karma will just go its own way and end without suffering the consequences. I am saying, 'O.K., we have a physical body but then there's the spirit part.' But for most people it is very difficult to see beyond the limitations of the physical body. Their thoughts are entangled with physical matter. That's problematic when one's existence is mostly spirit with karma.

"Then is it easier to understand or accept oneself as basically spirit when one is not trapped in a body?"

If a cultivator frees his or her spirit from the body then the true nature of existence is seen. But in a uncultivated person, the spirit that leaves the body carries or goes on with its own karma. It carries on—it's still confused. That existence is more like a total dream state. It's like nothing is in control. Whereas in a live body, there's an ego that actually helps to control the karma and its manifestation.

"But suppose a person already transited is now in spirit form. Perhaps the spirit hangs around—people dream about their relatives who have died. And they feel that their close departed relatives are there helping in invisible form."

I think in this context, most of the dreams are just memories of the dreamer. In actual fact, the departed deceased person could have been transformed and could be anywhere else.

"The spirit is not hanging around?'"

No—it's just the memories or the energy of it. That means when certain conditions are ripe, they can be retrieved and seen in energy form and the entities have intelligence like any form of energy.

"Well that makes sense—recently CNN interviewed a fellow who claims he can sense and converse with the spirit of the departed. Perhaps he's not talking to anyone but just sensing the energy of the questioner."

This psychic may have special training or gift to be able to pick up that kind of vibrations and energy from the person. According to Buddhism, the spirit or karma leaves the deceased totally from the physical body within seven days of death.

"Is karma something that can only be released from a human form?"

If the transition takes place, and the person is reborn into animal form that itself is just a specific manifestation of the karma. The remaining karma that follows will all be latent within the animal form. That means it will not be fully played out in the specific form which is a small fraction of the total karma. That form could be followed by another animal form, or a 'deva' or angelic form. It's all staggered— depending on the layer of the karma and it's layers upon layers again after that.

"So it doesn't have to be rebirth in physical form then?"

No, in the spirit world or the world of the departed on the seventh moon, according to Chinese belief, they will come out. But even that belief can create that kind of spirit entities. If a person expects that to happen, upon departing, at a certain period of time he actually has to transform himself into a spirit that comes out begging for food. What I'm trying to say is this: The playing out of karma can take place in any kind of existence—physical and nonphysical.

"Does freeing oneself of karma occur in human form?"

Otherwise you suffer the consequence. Once those effects are endured completely, then its over. For example, a person is reborn as a dog—so he receives his punishment. It may get bullied around, thrown out on the street, eventually it dies from hunger. That is all its karma—pertaining to that dog's life. Yes, all these animal forms act on instinct or in a dreamy state in some other forms. They can't be actively involved in freeing the spirit. Only in human form is it possible to unwind karma. So the human form is very unique. Even existence as a deva or demigod is just a dreamy state. That means you're not in control of what is happening at all. One cannot actually change it.

"Is this the only world where it's possible to do it to free yourself of karma?"

Apparently so.

Pure Heart

"But why is this world so special but still full of suffering?"

Without suffering, you'll never go ahead and practice. Probably there are other planets where complex human-type life exists. So perhaps there are other places, but humans are still a special form—free thinking, free creation, and also free destruction. Freewill and choice all happen in this form. So there's choice to create even more karma or get rid of it. All other forms—it's live and let live. It's playing out the previous conditions as in other forms the element of Heart is not there. There's no Heart—it's instinct.

"Say again. Sometimes I understand what you mean by Heart. Then I get confused by its meaning in other contexts."

The Heart is where one's innermost intention is. It's located in the physical heart area but it's not the organ itself.

"What is Pure Heart?"

In the human form, the energy or psychic Heart is located in the same place as the physical heart. In there, all the tensions and knots all are linked to it. In meditation, eventually you have to go in and free it outward. When you free it outward, it causes complex changes all over. One is totally freed—it merges with the pure energy. That's called the cosmic Heart itself.

"Most of the time when you refer to the Heart you're talking about the psychic Heart?"

Yes, but in cultivation, we're not going to concentrate on this. I mean, although we mention so much about the Heart, in practice it does not mean we are going to concentrate in the region of the physical heart. That itself will create tension. We are talking about the letting-go concept whereby the lowermost part of the torso—that's the lower abdomen—will ensure that the tension trapped in the body, including the psychic Heart itself, is properly released.

"So it is indirect?"

We can't work directly on the psychic Heart—It will mess you up.

"So the psychic Heart is not the Pure Heart?"

The psychic Heart has karma. It's laden with all the burdens and impurities. But when you talk about the spirit—that's pure. Spirit refers to a very vital vibration whereby a person exists. Because of the spirit you exist. It is vital vibration—whatever a person is.

"Spirit has no identity?"

It's already loaded with all kinds of identity of a person. But once the spirit is freed then it becomes pure Spirit and that's equivalent to the state of Godhood or Buddhahood.

"So again there are two kinds—ordinary spirit that's loaded with identities that when cleared off will then reveal the true Spirit?"

Yes.

"So the spirit is the life force?"

Yes, it's the life force itself and the spirit is full of identity. This identity means that it has karma and tension.

"What's the difference between the psychic Heart and the life force?"

The psychic Heart itself is the main control of the Spirit—the vital vibration. The Spirit can be huge, or tiny, or it can be everywhere. So there needs to be a control and that's the psychic Heart.

"Is that the equivalent of the brain?"

Yes.

"Except it is not the brain itself?"

It's not, haha.

"There we go—another layer of confusion for people who believe in the supremacy of the brain. Why does the universe makes things so complicated? Can't win—maybe one per cent can make sense of this."

True, one in a million.

"Or the hexagram of the Book of Changes will say-one in ten million."

That's the cosmic joke! That will ensure that existence or life will be continuous. Otherwise, if everybody understands the riddle of life—there's no more show, there's no more existence.

"Or soap opera."

In the end, there's no living humans. Fin. All become pure spirits.

"Infinity will disappear with no infinite time left. That's a similar notion espoused in atomic physics. There's radioactive material and in their half-life, half of it will be transformed to pure energy. But a half is sometimes hundreds of thousands, even millions of years. And what's left has yet another half-life with millions of years—and then there's a quarter left and this is repeated to infinity and infinite time."

More zeros than you can count!

"So going back to pure energy is endless. Another thing that's perplexing—there's pure energy and there's the energy that holds the atoms together. The latter energy is within some matter or called a specific element. Is such energy different from pure or cosmic energy?"

The energy in the atom is literally the identity—it has been identified with the atom and its structure. So it has become a rock, plant, or human in form and has been so identified. Once you remove the identity, the energy is undifferentiated. In terms of the cultivator it's the same thing. We are identifying the energy with the person or the tension of the person. If we fully reduce the tension or the karma or their identities, then it becomes or goes back to pure energy. But in this person now existing as a spirit it then becomes a pure Spirit.

Put it another way—it's dangerous to identify enlightenment with pure energy. Pure energy in quantum physics may not be the same as pure energy in enlightenment. Humans have a unique existence but once purified then it's certainly different from freeing the identity from a rock. A human has a previous existence in a human form.

"So it's not correct to say that the pure energy of atoms is the pure energy of cultivation?"

It's not the same. The difference is that there's a pure consciousness involved. Atomic energy has no consciousness. It has identity only but without consciousness. There are similarities, but its existence is purely electro-mechanical.

Part 5:

Return to Penang, Malaysia

6

On the Transparent Self

"Sifu, it is good to be back to see you again before heading home to Canada. Since we last met, I have read of some Canadian research attempting to show that prayer has the power to heal patients who are hospitalized."

Although prayers work, most people don't really understand why. They may feel that all their problems can be solved this way. But all that really happened is only a temporary solution to their presenting problem. They don't know how to seek more permanent solutions, nor do they really care. Whether they are ill or aging, they blame others for their troubles. When they are sick, they seek the help of a physician or a higher being to cure them. Most people prefer not to know the origins of suffering or the true cause of their problems. So when they age, it's the same. They may blame others or take it out on people.

Make sure that you are clear about cultivation. Ultimate benefits or results come from your own efforts and cultivation. In the words of the Vajra Sutra that says, 'All methods and all ways practiced are but dreams or bubbles, like clouds and mist. It's there for the time being but disappears when the sun rises.' Or it is just the reflection of the moon in the water or flower in the mirror. You are entitled to enjoy it, but remember that it's unreal. So eventually you have to go into it—the principles of purity, to seeing the real moon and flower. So you are entitled to enjoy, to admire, but make sure you don't indulge.

Cultivation of a Wisdom Path

"I do notice you are very slim, your hair seems darker, and there's more of it. Is that what you mean about reversing aging?"

What is the optimal reversing? We are referring to optimum functional ability of all the cells in the body. That is the ideal stage. That is the perfected stage. That means the body reverses back to its optimum. As an adult we are already well into the deteriorated state. So go back to the optimum state. Optimum means all is perfected. Physically, and mentally in terms of attitude there is no attachment and spiritually there's no more karma. And that itself is already the enlightened state. But for most people even in their prime state of health there never was an optimum state. We are born with all the imperfections.

"This optimum—is it standard for everyone or does it vary with each person?"

All Buddhas who have become perfected ones will look alike. In the optimum perfect state of energy, there is a constant likeness. There is no longer any mental identity or attachment and no karmic load on the Spirit.

"So that's a complete clone then?"

Yes!

"But as you mentioned we are born with a lot of imperfections. So that isn't reversing because even going back in one's earlier life span, there was never a time in the past that one was truly healthy?"

Correct. It involves reversing the process, but more than that it is also an improvement. So reversing the process of aging is not to an original condition.

"Tell me more—What is this optimum state?"

Truly, you feel you are one with the cosmos energetically and spiritually. One doesn't feel a self as distinct. The physical body is here but at all times you don't feel you are important. It's not there! The body, in terms of physical sensations, feels so loose and so light. You are virtually not carrying the weight of your body. Mentally, you don't feel compulsive of any thoughts or concerns. Stray thoughts don't arise at all.

Thoughts are functional according to the conditions you are in. There are no stray thoughts. Thoughts occur as a necessity to deal with conditions. If not, nothing arises, like a pond's placid surface that is totally ripple-free. The mind-spirit initially is like water in a pond murky with much turbulence.

"Yes, the mind is routinely peppered with stray thoughts, some conflicting, making it turbulent indeed. So cultivation of a wisdom path like Tao changes that."

Now it's totally cleansed. The water settles and is totally still. But still water does not mean that it will not be stirred and influenced by, say, wind or a pebble falling in. Make sure it is totally still so that only when the wind blows will ripples appear. When the wind is not blowing let no ripples arise. There's no turbulence anywhere. Only the turbulence in the moment.

"What is the purpose of the optimal state now that there is no more identity?"

It's a transcendent state. You feel totally at ease. You feel joyous at all times. No problems will arise.

"How does that help the world?"

First, even the process of cultivation itself helps others. Metta is created. In order to cleanse your karma you create the Metta. So the karma is diluted and goes into infinite space and time. The ancient traditions have such a belief. If one member of the family becomes a monk seeking enlightenment, seven generations of descendants will benefit. That is an attempt to describe how important it is to follow the path of cultivation. In the Taoist context, once a person reaches the Tao, attaining the ideal 'sien' state, or advanced state of cultivation, even if one stops, animals or chickens living in that environment will also reach sien-hood. That is, they will also evolve higher. It implies that all those around the advanced cultivator will receive tremendous benefits. That's a reciprocal chain effect.

"That is true since all energy is connected, and purified energy in one person radiates to all."

On the Road to Enlightenment

"Come back to CFQ and its effect beyond physical health."

Most people when they think of spiritual ascendance or development, are thinking of certain benefits—like peace of mind and contentment.

"We're talking of certain types of emotional states, isn't it? That should be very healing—since they're the opposite of depression. Feeling depressed leads to anxiety, tension, etc.."

Yes, that approach is certainly not wrong. But the peace of mind is a created state—that's what most religions refer to. It's a created state of happiness. But we're saying no, you don't create it. Rather, you adopt the let-go approach and that will loosen and melt away all the negative emotions. Those negative emotions are the karma, which is the cloud-like, sticky stuff. Once you melt them away, then you naturally develop the joyous state. Of course, this is peace of mind itself—but it comes naturally.

"So it's what's left?"

Yes, it's what's left. It's not what should be created.

"But how often can you get to the joyous state? I'd like to have more of that!"

It depends on how well you're cultivating. Of course, that state is infinite and that means it doesn't stop at any particular point.

"It's not an all or none state?"

It's not, it's hindered by our karma. The hindrance center is the karma itself—the dark clouds. When you remove it you get the joyous state.

"I imagine there's so much to remove that there's always another layer after that. So you have to get through each layer before you can experience the state again?"

Yes, the perfected state is when you've cleansed your karma totally and that is the Enlightened state.

"Is the joyous state then permanent?"

Correct.

"And not before that?"

Before that you have a piece of it.

"In your own case, do you feel you are getting more and more of that joyousness?"

Certainly, yes.

"How is it different as you go along, in terms of how you would describe the joyous state?"

Each time the feeling is not the same. It's something that's indescribable—it's there.

"What about features like intensity, can it knock you out?"

I did have a very intense kind of feeling—and that occurred a few times including the time I had my so-called occult initiation—the revelation.

"Yes, I remember very clearly the three initiations you had into the wisdom state of intuitive knowledge that revealed to you, for the first time, the CFQ mantra and your whole energy healing system."

The rest varied in degree—but you can recognize it. Each is not totally the same—well, the physical world itself does not bother you. In fact when I go into my meditation, most of the time even with the karma and clouds present, they still don't bother me much. That is a state of peace. Nothing matters.

"But do you still wish to move on faster?"

No, as you go further you understand more about the nature of karma and you don't get impatient. Patience is necessary and you go along.

"Describe those layers of karma. You mentioned them previously in general terms. What are they—thoughts and memories?"

No, most of the time you physically feel them as glue in you; glue that is melting off. The body gets stiff because it's affected by the glue. There are layers and layers—the body becomes very deformed in energy pattern. It goes beyond you like a cloud extending beyond your body's physical boundaries. It gets melted away; it leaves you and also has particular information.

"Is there a conversation going on?"

It's just like reading it.

"Hmm—what is it, is the information about your children, past experiences? What kinds of things?"

It's whatever occurs. Sometimes it's past experiences—like shameful things you've done. Or knowledge, or minor issues, or good events that have occurred in life. Some of it is like reading a story that doesn't seem to be too relevant to you. Some are your emotions. So it's all kinds of things. Anything can come in within the area of imagination itself.

But now you know that this is not imagination as you experienced them. You allow yourself to be unmoved by them—I mean, you must at the same time make sure you're with the Mantra. All the time, you stay unmoved by all such things and thoughts and emotions. If you choose to stop the Mantra you will straight away move into the emotions. Avoid them as this way you can even unconsciously be talking about this information or acting out what is suggested or even perform what occurs.

This is in line with what I mentioned to you before. When you do the meditation practice you made use of it to analyze your thoughts. Of course it's full of valuable information. You have by choice selected the information that is related to your job to give you fresh ideas. These totally fresh ideas are actually from your karma but they don't normally come because they are well-hidden elsewhere. The normal sense of thoughts are very superficial, but now are going deeper.

But these are still thoughts, still karma. Thoughts are from karma. You are allowing yourself to be a party to these ideas—you don't see them as your karma. But to be properly detached, just repeat your Mantra. Put on your unmoved Heart. Then you find you can literally see that all these are forces driving these ideas around.

The Incredible Lightness

"As a starting point isn't an intention for self-realization necessary? When one recites the Mantra isn't that the intention to connect with good energy—to the Mantra?"

As you advance deeper into meditation you are going into the spiritual aspect of who you are. Here it is no-intention that matters. To be sure the Mantra is to be spoken but ever so mildly. The intention is so mild that it is literally not there. It's always the understanding that matters, not the intention.

"What about the intention to let go?"

It's the understanding that one should let go, all right? We talk about the benefits of letting go. Once that's understood, just go ahead and do it. No more intention.

"In terms of mental thought, perhaps someone thinks about something missing in their life. So one's intention is to find what that is. The intention indicates one's interest."

We are all confined to certain patterns of thoughts. We are filled with our past experiences, our life pattern. To start something, there is always some intention about doing it. But as you advance further into spiritual development, it is without intention. You begin with the intention to go in. Then you gradually take away or melt that intention as well—Just do it! Meditation for the purpose of doing meditation is no longer good meditation.

"Then it has to do with faith—you just do it and that will meet the goal or your intention?"

Yes, in a way you can say we have to rely on the faith to carry on. But we are not talking about blind faith. In everything we need to do— even taking medication for an ailment, the element of faith should not be neglected. But in the path of energy meditation, you have been given an understanding of certain principles and you have also experienced certain phenomenon happening during meditation. Once these are made clear to you, you can drop any intention. Even the element of strong faith should be done away with then. The meditation should be without any preconditions and expectations.

"What typically happens during advanced meditation?"

You will see how the body changes. I am in the state where most of the cloud-like forces are already loosened. I'm in the folds—I'm fully aware of the folds in the body that extend outward. These folds and chunks are the impurities, the physical existence, the karma. Beyond that, there is this total transparency, the radiant Pure Light that goes out to the eternal, that fills up all known space. One can deny its existence. But no, it's there and it can be vividly experienced. It is alive! That is Me that exists without boundaries. That is the extended energy body—boundless and unmoved in all situations. It has no likes or dislikes. It is compassionate and will readily help. It is the pure energy of the Mantra.

"What's the difference between chunks and folds?"

Chunks and clouds are very thick. Of course, each time you melt off some tension, it converts into a cloud. But as the purification process goes on deeper, then you encounter only the folds in the sense that the melting away process is so fast you don't see the cloud anymore. The whole body is literally very folded and these folds come in every imaginable form.

"Folds mean forces that are more compact or dense, and chunks are bigger?"

The chunks are converted from the glue. What creates the folds is first the glue. The glue pulls back and then it's the folds. If you dilute the glue it becomes chunks of forces that can stretch far out for miles. As the purification process continues, you're aware only of the folds because each time each unfolds and is released it's an outright purification. The time to convert the glue into impure forces and release them does not take much time—it's almost immediate.

"So the folds are the chronic accumulated tension?"

Yes, it's all physical. So when I move them out, my posture can be seen to change accordingly. In the process of shifting, I'm fully aware of the folds within. The bundles of it has got to change as you go along. The folds are everywhere and I am aware of all as I spread my awareness. You see yourself separate from the folds. I am nowhere. Once the consciousness is spread there is only the difference between purification and non-purification. What is already purified and what has yet to be.

"But it fills up your whole horizon?"

Oh it does.

"So all one's experiences are displayed?"

Yes, it's a full display.

"So it's like you're looking at a screen that's three-dimensional since you're right in it?"

Yes, you're not separate from the screen. You're right in it—so you're feeling it. You can go in and play around but because this fills up all space you're not moving in and out. As soon as you're conscious of it you're there.

"What do you do in there?"

Just keep the Mantra on. Just allow what needs to happen take place. You don't have any specific intention to clear out something. No, as you cultivate you don't do that. We know the interconnection of all forces and what is apparent here is hidden elsewhere under another spot. So it's impossible to say, 'I clear this'. That's just the tip of it buried deep.

"It's not only perception or seeing?"

You sense the thoughts and experiences information behind them. You see a particular fold—but it also has meaning.

"Does the meaning come by itself?"

Yes, you need not try to find out. The meaning comes to you—there's no need to analyze. Plenty of meaning comes to you.

"What's an example?"

Messages of particular events in the past stored in memory. They may be actual or imaginary events—there's no difference. The mind doesn't differentiate between them as it's all kept and stored. Our consciousness can sometimes differentiate—but over a long period we get confused between an imaginary or a real physical event.

"Is it a reliving of the past?"

Not exactly—the thoughts of the past experiences have been assimilated and stored according to their specific function. They've been sorted out and organized, but not according to a real sequence.

"Probably like a computer—in different files according to topic, for example. Once you release it, is it gone?"

In the totally purified state—yes. You go in and you are totally transparent. You feel absolutely no hindrance. You must really feel that—you fill up all the space without any hindrance.

"But how does it work through?"

"You've got this stored memory that's organized in folds. You see something physical; there are messages. Once you experience part of these, they are released?"

All right, yes.

"And so you don't have to bother or deal with them anymore?"

Correct. You will not be bothered. The beautiful part is that the memory is not lost completely. It's still somewhere there in the purified energy. Except that it does not bother you.

"Not bothered means it's lost the identity part?"

No, it does not become a compelling thought. You've let go, but you can consciously retrieve it. It's still somewhere there—but it's loosen—and has lost the tension or folded texture.

"So that means in the past that fold has bothered you?"

You may have forgotten about it, but it's there and by focusing on it this way, it's no longer a problem for you. There's no total erasure of it; you remember, but compared to the past there's no anxiety about this event. Now that it's released you can even laugh about it when you talk about it. You're not trapped by it.

"Does that mean the folds are all painful, negative memories?"

The thicker the fold the stronger and more uncomfortable the original experience. It comes within a lot of sensations—pain, numbness, heat, cold, etc.

"Does that mean positive experiences do not have much value?"

They don't cause pain or very little in contrast to negative tension. True, they don't have much impact, especially on the negative aspect of health. That's why people prefer to have positive experiences. It's the negative aspect that's sticky. So there's no need to let go.

"Just by the intention of letting go of these negative memories...?"

No, we are not intending to let go. We are just using the Mantra to apply the purification process. The moment you go into it, the Mantra itself serves as the purification process and through that what is impure is automatically displayed in the dilution process. Of course, when you unwind the pain, you feel the pain. But the reward is that the pain does not bother you anymore. That's the natural reward—not magic at all. You can get rid of it—the pain that was there before has gone. Then it doesn't bother you anymore. Most people won't come to this stage of knowing. They can't identify it. A painful memory is only a concept in the mind to them. They talk about mind or what they conceptualize about it all the time.

In my CFQ practice I am learning more about the glue. I have more in-depth knowledge about it—the whole body becomes bundled up by thick layers of forces. These forces are very greedy and are constantly drawn inwards in the acquisition process.

"You are referring to your meditation?"

Yes, these forces are experienced in meditation. But I am almost cleared of it, you know. At any moment when I go into it, I feel totally transparent except for these forces. I feel the body is deformed where the forces are not totally cleared out. All these forces are in folds, and are physical and have got to tear off from the body. It's very, very physical. It's all over the body and deformed beyond imagination. The entire body becomes deformed in meditation. Things burst out in a funny way—very strange indeed. These forces, with all the information that accompanies it, have different colors and different shapes but they are all in fact physical. They cause problems as they have manifested physically and they have glued onto the physical tissue.

"Do you try to release them?"

Yes, by way of the Mantra itself, so that sufficient merit is given for it to be melted away.

"Do you still do movements?"

The body will still tilt and move about slightly in different positions. It's a slow re-alignment of the body. The whole body becomes aligned. At the end of it the body is loosened as the physical tissue becomes very light. And this is not only during the meditation itself. Even out of meditation, the body parts remain loosened and become lighter and it's like there's no obstacles in those body parts. It is totally loose without obstacle.

"What about your mental state?"

It is very clear and the whole thing hinges on the forces themselves. There are some dream-like feelings but the dreams are just informative forces within the tension. Yes, the tension has all kinds of messages, images, etc. These are stored within the forces—they are like electromagnetic fields capable of storing information. They are meant to be released.

"So in the totally purified state it is completely pure and completely loose?"

One is literally the cosmic. These days I feel more and more clear even in the times that I am not in meditation. The whole thing seems to be very clear, very transparent. But the helplessness of life is also felt because I am not totally perfected. Helpless because things are so near and yet so far away.

"What is this transparency?"

During meditation, with radiant energy you are also looking out from the body. I find that the whole body becomes transparent except for those tension forces that have not been cleared.

"The body is radiating?"

Yes, as it radiates it becomes transparent. It's no different from anything else but all the material objects in the whole surrounding area becomes totally transparent. You are not isolated then as everything becomes transparent as well. So body boundaries are not there anymore. Ah—no more body boundary.

"Everything is just incredibly light?"

Yes, everything is light except for the karma. In the meditative state, when you feel the karma it is totally physical. It is deformed and is comprised of multiple folds and colors and information. All these will stand out as obstacles. Other than this, it is all totally transparent.

"It must be a very strange feeling then?"

It is absurd! But it is a very real feeling. You are now just that deformation. But the essential part of you is that you are just the environment. You are in the selflessness state. That is the ideal state, the Buddha state in Buddhism. In Buddhism, selflessness is not only in terms of actions or thoughts but also there is not a physically personal existence.

"This must be enlightenment. So you are now part of the wall?"

Yes, you don't have an existence. You're so loose that there's no personal identity.

"But are you still aware?"

Yes, you are fully aware and still know what is going on. In fact, the awareness becomes too clear. You don't exist yet the awareness is very clear.

"What happens to all the objects and things that are present in the environment?"

Those things are still all there, but you don't exist. There are no personal likes or dislikes and no attachment to anything.

"Do you become say—part of the tree outside?"

Oh yes. You see yourself become part of everything but you can tune into some object—so you are the tree or you are whatever is there.

"You can sense what it's like? So what does the tree feel like?"

It's almost as close as touching the tree. The tree remains the tree. It's just there. You tune in and you become the tree.

"What else feels different from your normal self?"

Let me see—you are in the meditative state so you're not concerned with how the tree feels. It's like things are all what they are, as is.

"They are just there, huh?"

Uh, it's just there, all right? You're not segregating the tree from the grass. You tune in and you are the tree, and as you tune in your body becomes more and more like the tree. It takes the shape of the tree and seems to have the consciousness of the tree.

"What about people?"

Once you tune into people, you get to feel their emotions, or their helplessness—that's all. What I feel about most people is that they feel totally helpless, just an entanglement of a ball of forces.

"In that state of transparency, you also feel the dense part of yourself?"

Yes, that is the problem because that's the unprotected part of you. That is a hindrance, an obstacle to total and complete tuning in. If you want to tune in there, you will also feel your imperfections at the same time.

"So what is enlightenment then?"

Enlightenment means being totally karmic-free; that means absolutely no tension at all. Because when there's no tension, there doesn't seem to be an identity. There can be a continual existence since there is still the physical body. Because now that you have cleared away all the karma or the tension, the body that is left freely exchanges with pure energy. It doesn't pull in or draw in forces readily unless you allow it to do so. But even then if the body doesn't have capital tension, it doesn't get stuck in the body and you can easily release it.

"So why does the Buddha smile in enlightenment?"

First, the Buddha comes to the instinctive realization that things are as such but one hustles and goes round and round to search for it. Second, when an enlightened person is karmic free, the tension has left and there's no reason not to smile. You see, in an average person, the tension is very strong. In one patient I saw, the jaws are so tightened and clenched, it threatens to crush the teeth. It's difficult to force open the mouth. But as treatment continues, the tension melts away suddenly and the jaws loosen and physically drop.

Once the tension that is trapped and glued to the physical body is released, then the person will be smiling at all times. Because the body is so loose and moves so effortlessly. No more tension means no more identities in the body at all. There is no more you and I, you see. And there's no emotion at all. It is the karmic-free state comprised of pure vibration.

"At birth, what force is responsible that can be so powerful to attract the energy down?"

It's the tremendous amount of karma which will define the future course of the newly born. So even an infant is full of imperfections.

"Do you still use the Mantra?"

Yes, because things are not perfected. If I am perfected, I should be able to appear right in front of anyone I talk to even if the listener is speaking to me by phone from Canada, ten thousand miles away.

Mantra of Goldbody Energy

"I'm not sure whether I am practicing the right way."

Put your Heart into your Mantra and with the Mantra on be willing to let go and you're undoubtedly doing it the right way. As you go on, things will improve and the improvements will be more or less automatic. Sometimes you get entangled in some difficult layers of tension but as you persist with the practice, suddenly it clears out. You know what that is and how to deal with it almost automatically.

"There has been a lot of self-discovery in the energy meditation."

Yes, because we are talking of dealing with ourselves—of what we are, and all the combined experiences put together. The tensions peel off, and you can actually see them going off. As you go in, there's always two forces that interplay—the force of good that is spread about by the practice of CFQ and the Mantra itself. As well, you can actually see the forces of tension—the karma itself leaving.

"What triggers off the release of tension forces?"

The Mantra itself is a suggestion that it is good or pure energy. That's the meaning of the Mantra. We don't want the good to be an attaching good. That means we want to make sure that the good is the purest form and is non-attaching. Then it can be karmic cleansing. That's why we use the Mantra instead of saying 'Good, good, good.' That is enough to create a solvent to melt away the tension.

"But what triggers off the release of the tension?"

Oh, if you've applied enough solvent into a stain, it will have to drop off.

"So where does the solvent come from?"

From the Mantra.

"So it's not the movements?"

No, it's not. That's just the evidence that the dissolved stain is going out—evidence that the tension is moving out. When you claim to be letting go you must allow the movements to occur. Moving is a process of release.

"The movement is not the solvent nor is it the tension?"

They are just the physical release of the tension.

"So the movements is a by-product of the experience of the tension going out?"

O.K. yes.

"But the movements can be in many forms?"

Yes, accompanied by many past experiences that the person have acquired. Hidden tendencies are simply information or knowledge that a person have acquired or were taught to the person. Bear in mind that there is always an interplay of two forces. Somewhere in you, because of the good energy you are bringing through, you are automatically doing the right thing to help yourself in the release of tension. For example, the right stuff includes dancing, self-massaging, or slapping, or whatever movements spontaneously manifest.

"I notice that many of the movements are repetitious and rhythmic. Do these have a calming effect on the mind?"

Yes, feeling opening out from the spirit goes through the mind and out of the physical body. It's always continuously diluting and moving out. Spirit is the deepest and the furthest extension out is the physical body. We are talking about the karma and the karmic attachment on the pure spirit itself. The mind is actually a manifestation of how the spirit has got to deal with the environment or physical surrounding. Yes, the mind is in-between the spirit and the body.

"When the body moves around, the tension is being released. Does that calm the mind which becomes brighter?"

It's not meant to calm the mind. It is supposed to dilute away what's in the mind so that the tension is not compressing the mind. That makes the mind loose and non-attaching. All experiences that have occurred will remain as an experience or memory of them. But experiences can have different strengths of attachment. But now they have become less attached.

"I am trying to connect what you said with relaxation energy. Is relaxation energy the spirit, or part of the mind, or...does it go in and out?"

Relaxation energy is defined as the karmic cleansing energy. That means the relaxation must truly come out from the purification of the spirit.

"So what is this energy then? Is it something already within us?"

I'm afraid this feature is non-existence in the laymen's sense. To do this, it must actually come in with a full Heart and you must be willing to let go. Just the willingness to let go is a very unusual feature. We are all built with a distinct tendency to acquire and to keep drawing forces into us.

"So relaxation energy is just there in the background and one doesn't have to do anything. Just by releasing the tension forces the energy becomes evident?"

By releasing, there is actually an opening effect in terms of the physical. There's a melting and loosening of the karma in the spiritual and because of that the mind becomes freed from the entanglement of the compulsive thoughts. As a result, the physical body is also opening and loosening outward. That means the force in the body will melt away.

"And does the relaxation energy help in melting those forces?"

Yes, relaxation energy means that it must be able to melt away these forces in order for it be qualify to be relaxation energy. In all other ways, the ordinary way of relaxation whether taking a nap or holiday is not true relaxation in our sense.

"So what is true relaxation?"

Ours is the way we are doing it. That means to melt away the forces that cause tension. Tension is a real force, so we must deduct that force. The normal form of relaxation does not involve subtracting or removing the tension away. It involves doing something that is not considered tensed from a person's normal definition. People define ways of relaxing differently, for example, go to a night club or disco or work out in a gym that gives a sweat. That's what they call relaxation. The mind is normally so cooped up with tension that the person must also drive up tension in the physical body to balance it out—then he or she calls that relaxation. To us no, it's just a tensing up process.

"What about meditation though?"

In meditation you must first be prepared and willing to let go. Then you must do the right way or method of letting go. Otherwise, a person dwells in a state that is not true letting go and the result is, at best, close to dreaming or sleeping. Sleeping is also not melting away the tension or the karma.

"In Japan, when I mentioned the words of the Mantra in English, they instantly recognize it and say 'Shinzenbei'. This phrase refers to the god of education or to everything that's good."

Yes, since it refers to anything that's good we are no longer specific because specific goodness means at best it's just good karma.

"A Korean student refers to the three words as three virtues well accepted in Korea, 'Truth, goodness, and beauty' in that order and so very familiar to them."

They are used to intentionally narrow it's meaning to represent the most important values in life or philosophy. But basically it all means beauty.

"Yes, pure splendor! Or as the Romantic poet, Shelley, said, 'Beauty is truth and truth beauty. That is all ye know on earth and all ye need to know'."

Yes. The highest thought or the greatest good is associated with the purest energy which is necessary to melt away the karma. Good energy melts away the karma that is very negative, dense, and attaching. There's no other way for the karma to go off easily. In fact, it chooses to cling on to the person fast and hard. You just use the right merits to melt it off.

"In my mind, I still find it very hard to understand why it will work—how does the Mantra attract pure energy?"

O.K., there is verification that what is behind the Mantra is a code for perfection that itself is good enough. The mind tends to....Let me restate that. The moment you say the Mantra without thinking of what it means it is already associated with good.

"But how does that lead to, the ability...?"

Every thought is...All right, the truth is Life is a continuous process of drawing in energy through whatever actions, functions or thoughts one is doing. That's a continuous and natural process. We are all born and equipped with that ability. Every thought is a conversion of cosmic energy and drawn into a person. So is every emotion and every action and because of this natural process, we have got to be careful with our thoughts so that we minimize the negative energy that is drawn in. But this idea of being careful with the thoughts in itself is not good enough because once the energy has built up in the body it continuously wants to draw in more energy. That is its nature.

We cannot tell a person not to think because he will still go on having thoughts all the time. It's futile to tell the person, 'Don't think because it's the forces accumulated that is doing the thinking.' It's not the person that is thinking. For example, anger is functioning on its own. So is knowledge. The cognitions are functioning on their own. Because of our background knowledge we tend to think in certain ways in accordance with it. But this thinking process means that you continuously make use of the cosmic energy drawn inwards. This adds to the capital sum of the tension energy that is actually being excited depending on the topic of your thoughts. It is an automatic process.

By being attuned to the Mantra itself, well, every thought is a conversion of cosmic energy, all right? But you're tuning yourself to a purity (the Mantra) that is non-attaching itself but that is radiant.

"Right, nothing sticks in the transparent body. Just energy that shines through."

Bodhisatttva of Energy Healing

"The alternative of attachment is to be non-attached. Here that means to radiate?"

Correct.

"Once attached it becomes impure?"

Yes, but everyone is helplessly attaching and drawing in forces all the time. I am hard at work trying to cleanse away whatever attaching forces there are. Once the attaching forces are taken off, one is either a bodhisattva or in the enlightened state. Sounds absurd but I hope I am in the right mind. I can't even believe it but it all seems so real. Saying it out loud to you I try not to describe or dwell on this as it sounds insane. I just have to keep going at it.

Now it's easy. I go in right away where ever I am. In sleep, I try not to sleep but to be with the Mantra as long as I can. I can't describe it but it's really and truly physical. The forces that I encounter are all felt physically. The whole body is tearing out physically. When the muscles pop out grotesquely, any one can see this happening as they jump here and there. The muscles will be popping in a very frightening way to anyone else who doesn't know what it is.

"I saw the physical changes occurring when you meditated."

"But the problem is there isn't anybody else who has gone through the same process to compare or talk to."

Yes, but I am totally aware of what it is and know precisely what it means each time. Well who knows when the next Buddha will show up to tell?

"But you are the one who talks about the function of being a bodhisattva in CFQ, meaning that you take on the traditional vow. So you also have to figure how to help others too."

Yes, oh yes.

"How is that going to play out?"

That's hard. People can be very cold and that can be disappointing. The more you help some, the more they cling, and it's a bottomless hole that you can never fulfill.

"Nor would you want to. Filling someone up is not a metaphor I would associated with CFQ. It's emptying that matters!"

Helping them unconditionally, they become totally dependent and their expectations are too high. The moment they don't have that exclusive attention from me they get angry and envious of the attention given to others. This is that helpless feature of life. As society goes on it's heading toward self destruction. This process probably can't be reversed by others' efforts. Some, however, who have the right karma will work themselves out of it. Most will just follow the flow. That means eventually it's all mutual destruction and self destruction. In meditation, you feel totally connected and one with the cosmic. The meditation itself provides merits for others, benefits that according to the Buddha, is the greatest merit one can do for others—that is to actually meditate.

The other day, I worked on a cerebral palsy child whose parents were afraid that their child would never walk. After four sessions, the child got up and started walking. But unbelievably the father spoke out saying, 'Now he's walking because he's no longer lazy, that's why.' No mention that perhaps my work has at the least contributed to this change. The child was healed but they did not show the slightest happiness—No excitement or appreciation was shown!

But I will do more in future that will be much more impressive. I'm not ready to talk about what that is but they are in my mind for now. I feel the day or time is near when what I do will be completely unchallengeable. When I'm ready I will do that.

"One thing I can say—If your ability to heal is only confined to yourself, no matter how miraculous it is, it will not be accepted. What you say and do can only be believable when they work for others. When they practice what you say and benefit from it."

Yes, I understand the notion that I must impart it to all my students. Even my students who started out with me have doubts. They come having chronic problems, with walking or migraines and after learning from me those problems have gone for many years. But that happiness does not last. When their health is constant they think there are no further benefits. They forget that their original problems are gone. Now that they no longer have any severe problems they say the practice does nothing for them.

"What about premonitions? I know you don't make predictions and I suspect you see that as a kind of temptation. You don't dwell on that or use that to impress other people. But isn't that one of the gifts of having cleared the karma, that you can see clearly into the future?"

The future can be changed or created! You see a person without an apparent future. It occurs to you that the patient's case is hopeless. But since you're involved with the person, you should try to change that idea of hopelessness. That itself is to be emotionless, coming back to the question asked earlier. In meditation, what I see I don't remember too clearly—unless I try real hard to recall it. I don't prophesy the future since everything is in flux. I may try changing whatever negative that is perceived toward a positive end.

"But if you get a forewarning of something happening that's negative to your patient or student, do you actually tell the patient?"

This is the irony of the play of power—of psychic manifestation. You see a misfortune but do not get too excited by it. If you can try to forget about it, probably the misfortune may not occur.

"Oh, is that how it works?"

You take it as a wild imagination. Erase it—then that misfortune will not occur. You get yourself not to be attracted to it. Unless it is so strong and you find that it continues to linger. Then maybe your effort is not working properly. If you have done the right thing that could perhaps reduce the impact.

Instead of thinking—'Oh, I believe what I perceive and what must I do to avoid it?' In actual fact, there's nothing much you can do since whatever steps you take, it will still occur. At the physical level, whatever things you do, you cannot prevent something from happening.

A lot of such things happen during the meditation but I forget them after my session. I know these are happening but I intentionally don't remember. In fact, in the standard half-hour healing session many ideas have transacted—so much change of forces and all that. At the end of it, I don't even remember it because I can't afford to remember.

That's not my job—which is to purify the person. To remember is to retain. I mean to retain such negative forces—that means you're not cleansing it! It's like if you leave something on the blackboard that's because you wish to retain it—if that's what you want. That means something remains on the backboard. The board is not clean enough to write anything new. But if your job is to clean it up then you simply erase what's on the board.

I simply do my job and keep doing that, you see. At the end of it, there are all kinds of suggestions that are energetically seen but to us that's not relevant. There's still a natural automatic voice that says: 'Do your job!'

"I still would like to ask you how you envision your Center's work."

What I can tell you is this—the way we do CFQ seems to be virtually against everyone. The normal functioning pattern of a person inevitably leads to a complete life cycle of birth, aging, disease, death. This whole cycle is an acquisition process. So any suggestion, any idea, and action that involves acquisition, most people tend to be very happy with that. But in talking about the proper letting go approach as adopted by CFQ, we appear to be against everybody.

But we validate our theories with Buddhist philosophy and practice. For a human to become a Buddha takes many years—thousands of years even. The same for a Buddha to be born. So we accept this endeavor to be lifelong and beyond. But CFQ is here to stay amid all the hardships. But every job that we do brings tremendous merits. Of course, these merits can't be quantified in a tangible way. Spiritual things are not that tangible. But it's tremendous. We just have to do our job. CFQ has faced all the hardships encountered thus far and it will continue to survive.

"I think your work is doing better than merely surviving."

A lot of people do know what we are doing but how many are truly involved? It goes up like a pyramid. As we go on, their depth of involvement gets less and less. Some will just read about it. Others will do a bit such as attend a workshop or have some treatment sessions. Some will have a longer interest. Perhaps spend a few years doing it. You see, people with genuine interest are few in number.

But that is still sowing the seeds to, 'Let-go!' What the person hears about letting go to-day—well nothing clicks. But it is one of the steps for that person to actually let go in the future. So we just keep doing our work. There is a clash of forces as well as interest here. The prevailing force is acquisition. But there's some level of respect for what we are doing and at least they leave us alone.

"But you are in this healing mission for the long haul."

It is unfortunate. For example, even the Buddha failed. What the Buddha taught is actually a letting go approach but as it went along, very quickly it became an acquisition approach to acquire more wisdom, acquire more sutra learning, more power, etc. The Way has been humanly interpreted as an acquisition approach. That was never Buddha's idea. But that is the Buddhism that exists today where most people believe in the power of acquisition. Enlightenment is not an add-on process because with the slightest chance of adding, that process quickly becomes the predominant feature in the teaching. We have got to be very careful about this. Of course, there are some learned individuals, a very few, who actually understand what the Buddha meant and taught.

Part 6

After a St. John's, Canada Conference

7

Downloading CFQ Healing Energy

On returning to Canada, I presented a workshop on, "Eastern holistic perspective in deconstructing Health Psychology," at an international conference in St. John's, Newfoundland. Arriving home in Fredericton, the expected materials from Master Yap, in two bulky envelopes, had arrived. When I telephoned Master Yap in Penang, before leaving for the conference, he told me that he felt inspired to personally write and contribute something to add to the book's value. The first page of his writing described what had led to this inspiration.

"July 31st, 1999 is the 19th day of the 6th moon according to the lunar calendar. It is celebrated as the day that Kwan Yin, the celestial bodhisattva of Compassionate Love becomes an enlightened being. This year the date is doubly auspicious since it is also St. Anne's Day. St. Ann's Church in Penang on this day is filled with people from every religion—Christians, Buddhists, Hindus, etc. who converge on the church to offer prayers. The church, reputed for its visions of the Madonna, has for long been known to answer every prayer attracting the faithful from all over Malaysia as well as overseas."

"On approaching this day of great blessings during my meditation, I have a special sense of warmth and purposefulness. I felt divinely guided and I know what to write! As I write this, my body is pulsating with warmth and a wondrous energy that fills me up. (It also reminds me of another compassionate energy coincidence that Chok experienced in the ancient Basilica standing before the Madonna's sacred cloak in Mexico City). I feel engulfed in this blessing emanating from Kuan Yin bodhisattva and the Christian saints. Then alongside with the blessing, I feel this strong resistance—a thick crushing mess that came. My vision became blurred, I couldn't breathe, my hands shook and I could barely hold the pen down to write. Perhaps this is a psychic war between good and evil. I swear that I have never felt this before. Then it subsided and now I am able to write."

Message I: **On Reviving a Comatose Person**

It usually takes a severe traumatic shock for a person to lose consciousness and then remain in a coma. The trauma can take the following forms:

1. A sudden shock from an accidental injury or springing from an emotional nature (e.g., intense fear);

2. Infections causing a surge in pressure in the brain;

3. Under the chemical influence of drugs or alcohol that drives up pressure causing a surge in the brain that cannot come down;

4. Succumbing to disease or deteriorating health, e.g., stroke or heart attack.

The tension characteristics of a comatose person are:

1. There is a strong pressure built-up in the head pressing on the brain. In some cases, the brain swells, and there may be blood clot or bleeding.

2. Energetically speaking, the shock causes a sudden drawing in of tension, upsetting the energy balance in the body. The body-tension is abruptly raised to the upper body congesting the chest and head. Often, this produces in the coma patient characteristically twisted limbs, fingers, and toes or feet pointing downwards—as if the person is being hung up.

3. If no proper treatment is given, there is a gradual shutdown of energy and physical systems. It begins with the biological functions of the organs of the lower torso, moving upwards until the heart and breathing stops. Such deterioration, in some cases, may also occur very rapidly in a matter of hours. In others, it occurs over a matter of days while in a few cases the coma patient can hold on for weeks, months, or even years.

Emergency conventional medical attention is always necessary before considering energy healing. What can one do prior to the arrival of medical aid and life-support measures? Start with encouraging the person to hold on. Keep the person awake as much as you can.

In coma, the patient is normally mentally functional but it is a kind of dream-like functioning. The person is stuck in a dream of nightmarish proportions. The dream contents include the immediate events that cause the coma, past major life events, worries and concerns for loved ones, likes and dislikes, etc. Most of the time, mental activities get entangled in such dreams, alternating from one event to another. The person feels utterly helpless and struggles in vain to wake up. That drives more fear and panic in the person. Then there are feelings of loneliness—the external world is at a remote distance including your presence, even while standing right next to the person in coma.

The coma person can hear you, although not too clearly as you seem to talk from a distance, as if blocked by walls. Even if you touch the person in coma, he or she does not feel that it is real. The person struggles to move but the body does not respond or listen. Perception of the outside world and ability to hear you varies in proportion to the depth of the coma person's dreams. If deeply engrossed in these dreams or hallucinations, the person becomes totally shut off from reality, hearing and feeling nothing. The depth and contents of the dreams vary constantly changing the person's awareness of the outside world.

On What Not to Do

In all cases, comatose patients can be revived, and often it is not too difficult. But there are common mistakes made by people. The correct rescue procedure comes from tension reduction, i.e., de-stressing instead of boosting-up which is tension forming. Consider this scenario:

Jane receives word that her loved one is gravely sick and has fallen into a coma. The news itself sends her blood rushing into her head. She is flushed with anxiety and her thinking blurs. Her body is panic-stricken and stiffening. Jane rushes to the hospital like a torpedo. The very moment Jane sees her loved one lying in the hospital bed, she tries frantically to wake him up. She tells him to be strong, to will himself out of the coma. Jane actually shakes him and when he doesn't wake up she tries and tries again. Jane, in tears, also prays hard for a miracle. Gradually, her hopes dwindle and she falls into despair. As the days passed, she mechanically continues to visit him praying for a miracle to save him.

What Jane has done is putting tension into the coma person which can only result in further deterioration. Even though there are no physical signs, the person has probably been trying desperately and fiercely to revive himself. He is entangled in his attempts. He is too tensed up. If one tells him to be strong that will not help because he is already too "strong"—he is bundled up by the "strength" which refuses to let-go. If one tells him to will himself out of the coma, that is precisely what had happened—he willed too hard and set a trap for himself! You are causing more panic for him, and as he struggles even harder, he sinks deeper into the coma. Compare this to a fly stuck in a spider's web or a person trapped in quicksand. The greater the struggle, the deeper the entanglement and the faster it ends. If the victim had waited without struggling, and remained relax a way out is possible or help may come to free the victim.

The following actions are also not helpful in reviving the coma person since they will also put more tension into the person and cause deterioration:

1. The use of medicinal or 'brain' tonics aimed at nourishing and stimulating the brain actually raises the tension energy. Sometimes, even drugs to dissolve blood clots and induce circulation can be harmful. Of course, the proper use of drugs administered with professional diligence is necessary to manage the situation. Life support systems and emergency measures such as tracheatomy can help the patient to pull through.

2. Visitors talking aloud in the presence of the patient, often about gloomy predictions cause plenty of disturbance for the patient. Visitors presume that the patient can't hear them anyway but indeed he can. He hears, for example, that he may not have much chances of survival. Imagine how upsetting that can be!

3. You call in the priest or minister, or church members to pray for the patient. The patient interprets this as his last rites and farewell. Imagine how much despair you cause him!

4. You stretch his hardened joints, or you get someone to massage him, or an acupuncturist to work on him. The intention is good—to improve blood flow and circulation. But then his body may not take it. Even though most of the time, he can't even feel your pinch, at other times, his body can be very sensitive. The stretching, massage,

or acupuncture may cause so much pain that you throw the patient irreversibly all the way deeper into coma.

In fact, I know cases of conscious patients who are literally thrown into coma by such actions. Arthritic people, especially children, are vulnerable. If the therapist stretches such a person, the child may scream in pain and the therapist may think that this is just a spoilt child wanting to be pampered and continue the stretching. As the patient endures the repeated pain induced, the anger generated by the accusation, and his contrary protestations to the therapist being neglected, the child has no way out but to hide by falling into a coma. Post-stroke patients are also vulnerable.

Doing it Right

I have found that there are right ways of reviving a comatose patient. What I suggest below is not meant to replace nor interfere with conventional medical treatment nor pretend that you have the medical knowledge to treat the patient. It is simply what you can do what's right to help out or provide necessary social support to a loved one or friend.

1. First, calm yourself before you even see the patient. Breathe deeply and easily into your abdomen, I mean breathing with the diaphragm. This changes your tension pattern. A tensed person breathes heavily and shallowly with his or her chest. Remember the direction of the de-stressing procedure: Opening out from inside; flushing downwards and outwards. There should be no added input, only letting-go.

2. The first thing to do with the patient is to touch and tap gently on the lower abdomen, specifically the area just below the navel. Encourage the patient to breathe easily but deeply into the lower abdomen. At the same time, you should be doing the same. This area is traditionally called the 'Palace of Life.'

3. In between what you do above, comfort the patient. Tell the person to take it easy on himself or herself. Tell the person that he or she will be all right. Make sure you are not pressuring the person. All the person needs to hear is comforting assurances.

4. Repeat the above with patience and perseverance. Often, the person may not hear you properly or feel your touch. Keep trying.

5. Make use of the techniques suggested under the next section on 'Prayers and Energy Healing.' Connect and tune in to bring through CFQ energy. Even though you know nothing about healing, have full confidence in yourself.

6. At other times, talk to the person as often as you can. Talk about pleasant things and light issues. Do not create any worries or concerns for the coma person.

7. Touch the person as suggested below as often and as much as you can, even though the person in coma may not respond or may not be aware of your touch at all. Touching helps to sooth the person, removes the loneliness and sense of isolation from reality and from fear of the unknown. The touching can help to bring sensation back to the patient's body. A person's sense of feeling is normally strongest at the upper torso including face, head, and chest region. However, you should not concentrate on these places but rather lead the sensations downwards to the abdomen and legs. You can stretch and move the person's body and limbs as well. That helps blood circulation and brings back the patient's sense of touch. Take care not to be too forceful in loosening any stiff joints.

8. You may then observe that the patient's breathing has gradually gone down into the lower abdomen. By then, some coma patients could be out of their coma! Encourage them to breathe in and down lower—all the way down and out of their legs.

9. When the patient improves or has been revived out of coma, continue with these treatments.Use the CFQ prayer technique (see next section) to harness healing energy. Do not be discouraged by obstacles or swayed by negative suggestions. Subsequent progress in revival may have ups and downs but the treatment methods should be maintained throughout. You have done it right in the first place, so do continue the right stuff.

The CFQ way is one method for all problems but of course there may be limits to your success. The consolation is that despite not being an energy healer, you will have done such a great job! So be content, be grateful, and keep trying! Eventually, nothing can stop the patient from improving further and completely.

Chok knows of one comatose patient I have revived. The patient had 80% brain damage as shown in the brain scan. That patient was healed with all physical and mental functions recovered and practically no memory loss.

So I encourage you, if ever the occasion arises, feel empowered to help your loved ones or friends out of their coma state. It is comparatively easy to follow the CFQ way to release the tension down and out. Sometimes, however, after revival or once they wake up and can think again, things may not remain so easy. Someone might suggest another form of treatment and the patient may think this is more superior imagining a faster or miraculous cure. Fantasies are more appealing and they may doubt the CFQ approach. They begin to believe that such a simple treatment cannot be of much value. They wish for interventions that are more sophisticated or accepted by society. Then they may object to CFQ and their progress is obstructed. They selectively forget that just days ago, the line between their life and death was pretty thin.

Signs of Recovery

However, if you do it the right way, most coma patients will show some response within minutes of the first session itself. The patient's revival responses include eyes blinking, increase in eyeball rotations, swallowing, mumbling and vocalizations, grinding of teeth, coughing, change in breathing pattern from shallow chest breathing to deeper abdominal breathing, heavier breathing, facial expressions, increase in involuntary movements of body and limbs such as jerking, stretching, and shaking.

A combination of some of the above changes can occur at any particular time, alternating and fluctuating as the treatment progresses. Do not try to influence the changes. All you need to do is—Relax fully, and continue with bringing through CFQ energy, or patiently continue with physical soothing and verbal consoling. Check your own breathing now and then to make sure that you breathe all the way down your abdomen.

If you are the tensed or panicky type of person who can't calm down easily, find someone else who is calmer to do it. But the person must work with full sincerity. Staying calm and relaxed at all times while dealing with a comatose patient is most important. Sometimes, the patient may not be very sensitive to your words or touch but most sensitive to your emotional vibrations. That means, the patient literally can pick up your tensed vibrations. This is the most difficult area to handle since you are overly worried and affected by the loved one's life that is at stake.

The waking up process itself is normally gradual. However, in some cases, the patient can literally jump out of the coma. Some patients will dream-talk themselves out of the coma. Some may scream in pain before waking, with their body and limbs twisting in a frightening way. This is because of the unwinding effect of tension resulting in a cramp-like response. You need to assure the patient that he or she is all right. Tell the person not to fight with the pain and cramping nor to prevent or control it. Tell the person instead to let go, take it easy, and let the pain and cramp move their way out.

In the process of bringing through healing energy, it is also usual for the patient to show grieving and display painful expressions. These can result from the release of emotional or painful memories, or the 'tearing-off' of physical tension. Verbally comfort the patient. Verbally assure the person. Tell the person not to fight, or control, or hold back. Be easy and be willing to allow the pain to move out.

In cases where the damage is too great and there is no hope of revival, your treatment can actually help them to remove the 'holding strength' which is keeping them in the coma. In other words, they let-go in the opposite direction which is an upward surge. Life then leaves the body. This is also good in the sense that you shorten their suffering.

So to ensure safety in normal treatment, you are therefore advised to touch and tap the patient's lower abdomen. That is, you protect the 'Palace of Life'. The unspoken command is—Get back down and stay in the body.

When Not to Use CFQ

As CFQ treatment can, in reality, be very powerful, you need to assess the coma patient's chances carefully before deciding on such treatment. Do not use CFQ in cases when a patient does not have a future such as:

> * Coma in the advanced stage of cancer where the decay in the body is so great that it is no longer suitable to sustain life;
> * Damage to vital organs that are irreparable or irreplaceable;
> * The patient is too old and feeble so that even before falling into coma, the person's physical state is in very poor condition.

The above is to prevent the danger that you have inappropriately over-protected and revived the 'Palace of Life', and tied life back to a body that is no longer suitable for life to continue. In such cases, you prolong unnecessary suffering. That is cruelty. The better alternative is to strengthen the dying patient's religious beliefs. Remind the person to trust God and God will take care of him or her. But please talk to the person about the alternatives as:

> God heals you if your time is not up
> God takes you away if your time is up

With these alternatives, the person is more willing to trust God. With that the dying person forgets to cling on to dear life. The cause of clinging on is fear of death itself. When the person trusts God, the loved one dies in peace.

Evaluation of the Patient's Condition

The following information can be used to assess the physical condition of the coma patient. But remember they are useful only as a guide but not to draw conclusions on the fate of a patient. Conditions may vary and change rapidly from time to time so that even an expert can be confused by the physical symptoms described below.

> * Rigidity of limbs. The appearance of rigid limbs mean that the coma person is able to hold on to life. If other critical indications are at least fair, the person is not in immediate danger. If the limbs are completely limp, this means that tension has been completely absorbed and life is leaving going in the upward direction. The person is in real danger. If is person is only temporarily unconscious, he or she will quickly regain some degree of rigidity as consciousness begins

to return, normally within hours. For the person in coma to hold on, at least one of the limbs must have some rigidity. Otherwise, the energy in the muscles of the limbs is wasting away rapidly. If your intervention is successful, the person's limbs should gradually become rigid. Further improvements come when the rigidity then gradually dissolves away.

* Involuntary movements. These movements suggest that the person is being self-regulative. When tension builds up, release is evident by the person's limbs jerking or stretching. However, such release is normally insufficient for the person to wake up. If the coma person is being stimulated emotionally or physically, there can be increased movements. You should avoid doing this as it creates tension. If the person cannot deal with or release the created tension, the condition worsens. When CFQ treatment is done, there will be more involuntary movements, meaning a reduction of capital or stored tension.

* Yawning and coughing. Yawning is a good regulative action that often means that a patient is about to wake up. Coughing is also a good regulative action and should not be suppressed by drugs unnecessarily, unless the coughs are too violent and frequent.

* Eye movements. It means that the patient is mentally busy— either thinking, dreaming, or hallucinating. This is normally a good indication. Rapid blinking of the eyes means, for the worse or better, that there is a physiological struggle against an internal change. If the eyes are wide open and appear blank, it means the patient is probably deprived of oxygen. When the eyes rolls up, the person is completely suspended by tension in the head (from the situation above). If the eyes appear stale and lifeless, and do not even respond to a pencil light, the condition is critical.

* Tongue protruding. When the tongue sticks out, the person is squeezed by the suspended tension in the chest and throat. When the tongue rolls up, the person feels the suspension in the head.

* Facial expression. Varied expressions are better than a static, tensed expression.

* Breathing. Shallow, rapid breathing is not conducive to recovery. Your CFQ treatment should change it to a deeper, diaphragmatic breathing.

* Blood pressure. Stable blood pressure means the patient's condition is stable. Unstable condition is normally characterized by rapidly fluctuating blood pressure.

* Pulse. When the patient's condition is bad, the pulse is rapid, erratic, and it is often difficult to recognize a definite heart-beat.

Do not be overly disturbed by any adverse conditions you notice. Do not try hard to change them. Once you decide to use CFQ, relax and work according to the energy healing principles. Remember that you are not to directly change any of the conditions or symptoms you see! You are to zero into the life itself. That will change all adversities.

Message II: **Prayers and Remote Energy Healing**

Life is never short of surprises but when least expected the fates play their greatest tricks on us. One moment, life is marvelous as we soar to the greatest heights of our achievements. Success, when it comes is, however, seldom certain and the most faultless plans may fail without any apparent reason. Then there are the mysteries of life, of disease, aging, and death. We remain baffled as to where we come from, fearing the unknown future, and our own mortality.

To begin to understand life, I believe that all events are due to actions and interactions of unseen forces—the energies. All matter is variations derived from the one pure cosmic energy. Life is a function of karma—cause and effect. Uncertainties in life are a result of the complexity of such karmic forces. Many causal factors interact to come to a single effect. There is also the karmic forces of other individuals, that coalesce as a group or collective karma that then comes into play in an individual's life. Behind all these there is only one truth—a wondrous Pure Energy in absolute terms.

But there is also a human need to have forms that we can see, hear, and learn how to connect with. We pay homage to the departed saints and sages. We pay respect to past heroes and ancestors. We wish to remember them, aspire to be good, and we want some higher or greater unseen force to guide us on the right path. In times of loss and chaos, we pray to our merciful God, and even those who profess not to believe are brought to their knees. God is the greatest Good, The Almighty that nurtures life. And notice the word G-o-d. That's just Good minus one "O". Where has the other 'O' gone to? Out in the vastness of the cosmic! God cares and loves not only you-me but everybody.

If you have a different belief, that is perfectly fine. Let us not argue. Whatever your belief system, believe in full faith. Believe in utmost sincerity. We need a code of conduct, ethics, and a higher guidance to live in an orderly world. In times of great difficulties, one instinctively use prayer and pray to God for guidance and help. Even non-believers readily slip out the words, "Oh my God!" in adverse situations. God is suppose to answer. You wish that God will grant you your wish. Since God is Almighty, help comes to you and your prayers should always work. But you have doubts and you may be wrong to think otherwise! There may be good reasons why you did not get the answer you seek. Here are some ways you may want to check out to make a good prayer to ensure a solution to your problem:

* Sincerity. Pray from your heart. A half-hearted prayer is too weak to be fulfilled;
* Trust. If you don't trust God how can you trust Him to help you?
* Clarity of request. If you have not sorted out clearly your problem, you get confused answers;
* Single problem. If the many problems have been narrowed down to one, the answer may be unbelievably powerful. A critically ill person, who narrows down his problems to one gets a miraculous cure;
* Throw out your problem. After you have prayed, trust that God will help you. Throw the problem out of you. There is no need to carry the burden of remembering your problem. The burden belongs to God. You only remember your problem when you repeat the prayer. Repeat firmly only at specific times set aside for prayers. Do not repeat the prayer all the time. If you nag at God, God hears you not;
* Non-specific solution. Let God work out the solution for you. Give God time. Do not try to teach God what to do!
* Do no harm. God is fair and does not rob one person to give to another.

The answer to a prayer is totally in line with the law of karma, the cause and effect of energies. When one prays, one sows the seed to a solution. One throws out a problem and excites the karmic forces relating to the problem. Your request for a solution brings you a new set of karmic sequence.

Here, I offer you a way of using non-local CFQ energy through prayer. The easiest way of accessing this energy, without coming to see me, without learning about CFQ meditation, and enduring with such difficulty, is by means of prayer. Please do not interpret my intention wrongly. I do not have the slightest intention to be a guru, or establish a cult following, or elevate myself to the status of a God. I am saying I would like to share the results of my hard work on energy healing with you. I would like you to experience it. I would like you to benefit from it. I simply would like to help those of you who wish yourself, loved ones, and friends to be well.

Before beginning, I wish to say that I have a head, body, four limbs, and walk on two legs; that I have to go to the toilet several times daily—and I am as much a human as you are. But I have clocked over 35,000 hours in meditation, both in healing others and self-practice. That is equivalent to 18 years of a full-time job working 40 hours a week. I have worked on most types of known diseases and I know this—Healing energy works! And it radiates everywhere. It does not seem to have the ordinary constraints of space or time.

Praying in the New Millennium

Consider this as my personal invitation for you to try out, of course, with full sincerity:

1. Begin with praying to your God to permit me to bring through CFQ healing energy. God means the highest good according to your spiritual beliefs. By praying to God you remove the hurdle of disbelief to have sincerity and trust. To put it more straightforwardly, God heals you the CFQ way;

2. Relax on a reclining chair. Calm yourself and breathe naturally. Be mildly aware of your lower abdomen where the 'Palace of Life' is located. A sitting up position is preferred from lying down in bed as the CFQ healing path is by means of downward releasing and outward

opening. For a beginner to lie down, this healing path is not facilitated. If you stand, it is harder to relax.

3. Be open-minded and non-judgmental and be prepared to let new ideas flow through you. Be willing to explore new possibilities. You should not indulge in active thinking during prayer—do not follow your thoughts.

4. Loosen your limbs and rest comfortably. Be willing to 'open' your body. Be true. You should not be holding a glass of wine or doing anything else. That will distract you.

5. Submerge yourself totally in the blessing of God, just like dirty linen submerged in a tub of water. The difference—God's power is boundless. The tub has a thick boundary.

6. Within minutes, you should feel the healing energy flowing through you. Remain as an independent observer. Be non-judgmental. Do not participate in the activities of the healing energy. Do not try to force through a blocked passage. Let whatever be—As it is. Continue to trust God;

7. Be aware of your breathing becoming deeper and going down lower. Do abdominal breathing naturally.

At this prayer point, as the healing energy radiates through your body, you may experience a variety of physical responses. As you become more aware of your body, you hear your heartbeat, etc... If you close your eyes, you are more aware of the co–relationship of your body with the outside. You begin to see different shades of light, different degrees of darkness and brightness, different colors some of which you are totally unfamiliar with. You begin to see different lines, designs, shapes, and formations. Be non-judgmental. Do not tell yourself: 'This is my imagination.'

You may also feel tingling sensations in your hands, which soon spread all over your body. Feel the pulsations. Feel the improvement in blood flow. Feel your problems melting away. Feel how they get flushed down and out. Feel how they dissolve and dissipate. Get to know the depth. Feel how they melt and become numbed as they spread out on the skin and move away. You also feel other sensations—heat, cold, numbness, etc..

Allow your body to stay loose and relax. You may be aware that as the body tension unwinds, your limbs begin to twitch, jerk, and stretch on its own. Perhaps there are vibrations all over your body. This is the beginning of the involuntary movements. Do not be afraid. Let it continue to develop. Remain non-judgmental. Do not try to influence its course. Trust God.

As the unwinding process of tension release continues, a full series of movements unfold. You know you are not creating these movements. Your mind is peaceful and independent. Movements change in strength and variations. You may automatically get up to move. Be mentally non-participating. Continue to trust God.

Normally you should not restrain the movements. Just do it gamely and have fun. Unless the movements are morally unacceptable, do not try to change or control them. But this is highly unlikely. Energy has its set of rules. Unwind yourself from your deeper most psyche.

8. You may need to have the assurance of connectedness in prayer. Place this book against your abdomen, or on a table in front of you, or on the altar. This can connect you with the group CFQ energy field.

Find out much more. Discover for yourself. Explore and cleanse your spirit. Be willing to pour out your problems. Do this effortless exercise—Visually see your karmic entanglements. See your own thoughts.

Do the prayers and radiate the CFQ energy daily for one-half hour to one hour. You may experience an amazing sense of well-being. The benefits increase with time and regular practice. Some of you may fall asleep on your initial tries. Do not be discouraged. Just continue. Some of you may feel tense and restless. This is an initial hurdle but perseverance will bring the desired results.

9. You may want to do the prayer and go straight to bed. In sleep, you may have vivid dreams. If the suggestions from the dreams can reasonably be followed, just do it. If not, ignore them. If your dream suggests that you eat ten apples to cure your constipation problem, do it as it may turn out to be the solution.

10. When you wish to end your prayer, just tell yourself that you are coming back to the real world. Complete with a prayer of thanks. Walk and stretch yourself to feel completely back.

How can you use the prayer of healing energy? Think of doing this for yourself or others' well being. If you have any kind of health problem and seek a profound cure trust in God with your problems. Pray to Him to heal you. God helps you to come face to face with them. You get to understand them and watch them dissolve away. Of course, you get to see the mess that you were hiding from and may suffer somewhat as the symptoms are released. But it is worthwhile. Eventually you will get better. Meanwhile, you must continue to trust your physician. At the very least, the doctor can relieve you of your problems and help to control and manage them.

If you are critically ill, trust God as He knows exactly what is best for you. Let go and relax and submerge yourself in the blessing of God. It is now God's problem, and He gives you Peace and relieves your pain.

If you are visiting someone dear to you who is sick, you can pray on his or her behalf. Do it exactly the same way as you would pray for yourself, except that you must tell God that you are praying on your friend's behalf. Then relax with the understanding that you do this for your friend. Understanding means that you do not even remind yourself that you are relaxed on behalf of someone else. If you manage to establish good rapport, you may suffer the discomforts of your friend's problem. Consequently, however, you reduce your friend's suffering to the extent that you suffer in place of your friend.

Alternately, you may hold this book with one hand and touch your friend's lower abdomen with the other. You serve as the channel for healing energy which radiates to the patient.

Be careful not to try to use CFQ to revive a hopelessly critically ill person. If you prevent life from leaving a body that is not suitable to continue living you are doing a cruel act. Moreover, if the person eventually does not make it, the rapport you have created by trying to heal the person lingers on and may affect you adversely. In the unfortunate event that such an incident occurs, continue to pray to clear it out.

If you are requesting God to help your children in their studies, begin with the prayers months before any major examinations. Your prayers may initially cause temporary confusion and poor memory.

If you are looking for spiritual fulfillment, just pray for it. If you are interested to learn CFQ meditation, pray to connect you to CFQ healing energy. This serves as a good half-way bridge.

If you are a practitioner of other forms of Qigong, tai-chi, and meditation, and intend to find out about the CFQ method, pray for the connection. Through the unwinding effect, your initial attempts may reveal a strong manifestation of the old practices. Gradually, upon further thinning off your previous practice, you begin to experience newer understanding and experiences coming from CFQ healing energy.

If you are a healthcare professional, pray to discover more about the effect of non-physical energy on physical and psychological problems. If you are a scientist or a researcher pray to explore new dimensions.

If you are a homemaker and fed up with the monotony of household chores, develop a new hobby in communicating with God. If you feel fat, pray instead of sweating it out. You may lose weight faster. If you are underweight, pray and God will give you some weight. If you have career, finances, or family problems, try praying and see whether that can help you. If you are one of the very lucky ones who have nothing to request from God, just pray for fun or the joy of it.

I wish to invite everybody:

> Let us pray—
>
> For good health
>
> For a better world
>
> Letting go wholly—
>
> Be open, loose, easy
>
> Whatever it is—
>
> So be it
>
> Trust God to deal with it.

Epilogue

We thank the Enlightened One, the ancient Masters, our parents, and all our teachers in the path of cultivation. We are grateful to our temporal families who support us daily and our spiritual family for liberating us. We would like to thank you for your interest in this book. You have given us such a great opportunity to share with you what we know. We hope you have benefited from this book. We hope you try the healing techniques suggested and that they work for you. Those of you who practice or are interesting in Eastern healing arts, meditation, and Enlightenment may have experienced something more or different from reading the book.

I invite readers to contact the author to provide their feedback and comments. Tell us your experiences stimulated by the book, how it has helped, and what it has done or not done for you. What you communicate to us will help us to communicate further with you and others. Master Yap's final message to all, "Remember that CFQ Goldbody healing energy is available to you at all times. My sincere wishes."

CFQ energy healing brings true relaxation or Pure Heart energy for these benefits:

•Relax and let go to cope better, stay healthy, and resilient
•Relax wholly to be more able to help the sick recover
•Relax to help everyone else
•Relax and let Pure Heart help you.

About the Author

Chok C. Hiew, Ph.D., was born in Georgetown, Malaysia and moved to the United States in 1968 to attend the University of Colorado, Boulder. He is a professor of psychology at the University of New Brunswick in eastern Canada where he has lived since 1974. He has taught psychology and done research in numerous Asian countries in the Pacific Rim and has a life-long interest in meditation, Eastern healing arts, and psychological states of consciousness. His current area of investigation is on human resilience, holistic health, and longevity integrating mind-body psychology and Heart energy. The author's email address is: hiew@unb.ca